The Plant Paradox Diet

Eating for Health & Longevity

Zarrine Flores

The Plant Paradox Diet

Copyright © 2018

ISBN: 9781980421788

Warning and Disclaimer

Every effort has been made to make this book as accurate as possible. However, no warranty or fitness is implied. The information provided is on an "as-is" basis. The author and the publisher shall have no liability or responsibility to any person or entity with respect to any loss or damages that arise from the information in this book.

Publisher Contact

Skinny Bottle Publishing

books@skinnybottle.com

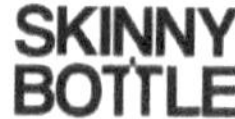

ZARRINE FLORES

Introduction

Thousands of years ago, long before laboratory facilities were available, people understood the importance of good digestion. So much so, that Ayurveda medical system claimed that it all starts in the gut. Many other healing traditions, including the Traditional Chinese Medicine (TCM), also emphasized that proper diet and good digestion are key to good health.

Unfortunately, in the Western culture, the importance of proper digestion has been neglected. Whether we allowed ourselves to forget the ancient knowledge or were deliberately encouraged to accept new ways of eating as normal, is a matter for discussion. Suffice it to say that materialistic worldview, busy lifestyle and government-prescribed diet focusing on grains, meat, dairy, and sugars, created the typical Western diet which is not only unhealthy but is directly linked to the so-called diseases of civilization: cancer, stroke, heart disease, obesity, diabetes and autoimmune diseases.

Not only is the typical Western diet difficult to digest, but problems that result from this diet, such as indigestion, heartburn, bloating and constipation, are treated with drugs, rather than a diet change.

Fortunately, this is beginning to change. As the world is becoming more polluted, and our food more toxic, people are becoming more health conscious and are beginning to look for ways to improve their eating habits.

The general trend towards a healthy lifestyle means that foods which are known to be full of good carbohydrates, antioxidants and vitamins have become the staple diet of those who want to do something about their health. And the first thing people are advised to eat when they switch to a healthy diet is whole grains as a source of essential nutrients, and beans and legumes as a vegetarian source of protein.

When Dr. Steven Gundry's book *"The Plant Paradox – The Hidden Dangers in "Healthy" Foods That Cause Disease and Weight Gain"* appeared in spring 2017, it caused quite a stir. It claimed that many of the healthy foods we've been deliberately eating to improve our digestion and general well-being, are not so healthy after all, and could even be the cause of many health problems.

It's not that we are not aware of the dangers that gluten can cause to those with gluten intolerance. What is shocking is that the main "danger" lurking in many "healthy" foods is lectin, a chemical found in almost all plants.

The philosophy behind *The Plant Paradox* is not new. Grains we eat today are very different from those available a thousand years ago, and gluten intolerance has been affecting more and more people worldwide. However, what the renowned cardiologist and heart surgeon Dr. Steven Gundry made us realize is that gluten is just one variety of a common, and highly toxic, plant-based protein called lectin.

To make things even more complicating, lectins are found not only in all grains but also in many fruits, vegetables, nuts, beans and dairy products.

Bookshops are flooded with diet books and nutritional guidelines, so you probably wonder if this is perhaps not yet another fad diet that the health-conscious and naive will fall for.

Dr. Gundry spent most of his career researching effects of diet on health and has managed to successfully treat thousands of patients suffering from autoimmune disorders, diabetes, leaky gut syndrome, heart disease and neurodegenerative diseases. His success lies in the treatment he used, which was to detox the cells and repair the gut. *The Plant Paradox* is the story behind this success.

We live in an increasingly stressful world where just keeping up takes a lot of energy (both physical and mental). To help your body cope with ever-increasing pressure and constant change, your immune system must be strong, so it can protect you from disease, as well as increase your chances of recovery in case you get ill.

According to Traditional Chinese Medicine, people can voluntarily increase or decrease the amount of energy (physical, mental and spiritual) in their body, creating, or destroying, the harmony needed for optimal health. There are different techniques of balancing one's energy, the easiest one being through diet.

A lectin-free diet will probably require some major changes in your eating habits and lifestyle, however, if you know that you are ensuring proper absorption of food nutrients and smooth running of your digestive tract, the switch won't be so hard to do.

In this book I'd like to encourage you to eat *a la Gundry* and, whenever possible, avoid lectin-rich foods. It's unfortunate that many of the foods known to be full of lectins are very healthy, so rather than give them up entirely, you should learn to prepare them in a way that will make them more digestible. There are cooking and preserving methods that can "tame" the destructive effects of lectins on your gut.

You will benefit from the Plant Paradox diet if you are lectin-intolerant, or if you've been suffering from a leaky gut, constant fatigue, bloating, gas, skin rashes, joint pain, allergies, nausea, muscle weakness, numbness, and particularly if you've experienced several of these conditions.

Your health and happiness depend on the state your body is in, so why not help it maintain balance so it can continue to serve you well. As Astrid Alauda so beautifully put it, "Your body is a temple, but only if you treat it as one."

PART 1

Chapter 1

When Eating Healthy is Not Enough

Eating healthy is as much about what you eat, as about your attitude to food, and the ability of your body to extract the nutrients from that food. In other words, healthy food can only be nourishing if it is absorbed and digested properly. How to help your body get the most from each meal?

Healthy Eating Habits

Our concept of eating healthy has changed many times over the past fifty years - and it continues to change. As science evolves and our understanding of nutrition grows, we begin to realize that what was considered healthy even only twenty years ago, is far from healthy. So much so, that even the latest government-issued nutrition guidelines are considered outdated.

As people become more health-conscious, there is an increasing trend towards a healthy lifestyle, which usually starts with a change of diet.

There are hundreds of diets which people follow for different reasons:

- To lose weight

- To gain weight
- For health reasons (to manage diabetes, improve cholesterol levels, lower blood pressure, reduce risk of heart disease, avoid certain allergies, etc.)
- As part of a lifestyle change

So, whether you eat for pleasure, health, or emotionally, a healthy meal should consist of natural food, nutritionally suited to your lifestyle, and be prepared and eaten in a manner that improves digestion. Only then can you hope for your food to be "thy medicine".

There are many ways to eat healthy, and this varies with regions, cultures and individual budget, but generally speaking, healthy eating habits are those that meet your physical, mental and spiritual energy requirements.

The Three Essentials of a Healthy Diet:

Nutrition

Importance of a healthy diet cannot be overemphasized. Not just to maintain a healthy weight, but because poor eating habits, and particularly the Western diet, have been directly linked to the so-called diseases of civilization: cancer, stroke, heart disease, autoimmune diseases, diabetes, and obesity.

A diet which focuses on processed meats, refined carbohydrates, and dairy, not only lacks the necessary nutrients needed for optimal health but will sooner or later have a very negative effect on your mood and overall well-being. There is plenty of evidence that unhealthy diet can even lead to depression, anxiety, and some other mental health disorders.

On the other hand, a diet based on fresh fruit and vegetables, lightly cooked meals, reduced meat, dairy, and sugar, not only contributes to improved physical health but easily improves your mood and lowers the risk of many serious health conditions. The "real" food provides nutrition that supports your physical, mental and emotional well-being.

Food which is processed, over-cooked or extensively treated with chemical fertilizers is not only less nutritious but is downright dangerous. Heavily processed food is basically "dead" and all it provides is bad carbohydrates and lots of sugar and salt to make it tasty. The only thing it will do for you is help you gain weight, become addicted and develop cravings for such food. Over time, it will slowly, but certainly, undermine your health.

5 Ways to Improve Nutrient Absorption:

Food combining

According to the food synergy principle, when certain foods are combined, they become much healthier than when consumed individually, e.g.: broccoli and tomato, avocado and tomato, honey and walnuts, etc.

Adding fat to veggies, rather than cooking them in fat

Fat is necessary because it's a major fuel source, but also because it helps you absorb certain nutrients, such as fat-soluble vitamins A, D, E and K. However, cooking in fat increases calorie intake, so the recommended way of getting the most from both good fats and vegetables, is to add fats/oil to vegetables (raw or cooked) just before serving them.

Avoiding alcohol during meals

Drinking alcohol during meals disrupts absorption of some nutrients.

Chewing your food well

Digestion starts in the mouth, with the help of enzymes in your saliva. Chewing helps the breakdown of food, so it reaches the stomach already pre-digested.

Look after the friendly bacteria in your digestive system because it is instrumental in breaking down your food and allowing your body to use the nutrients. Take probiotics either as supplements or by including fermented food in your diet, e.g. yogurt, sauerkraut, etc.

Good digestion

There's no point eating healthy food if your body can't process it or absorb the healthy nutrients from it. Both Ayurveda and Traditional Chinese Medicine medical systems stress that there can be no good health without good digestion. Digestion is helped both by the kind of food you eat, as well as by the way the food is prepared and eaten.

According to Ayurveda, if one's digestion were perfect, there would be no imbalances, and subsequently no diseases. TCM also claims that all diseases start in the gut. Both these medical systems recognized the importance of enzymes in helping our bodies properly digest the food and use all the nutrients. This is why healthy diets should focus on fresh, fermented and natural foods, as well as on foods that aid digestion.

Undigested foods or foods which your body for some reason finds unacceptable (e.g. poisonous or toxic) often induce vomiting, abdominal pain, bloating, diarrhea, or even weight loss.

Healthy lifestyle

There are many ways to eat healthily and regardless of which one you choose, the energy and nutrient requirements of an oil-rig worker will differ enormously from those of a teenager, pregnant woman or a laboratory technician.

Your lifestyle will determine whether you need more protein and fats, or vitamins and carbs. Besides, different seasons require different diets, so in winter you should eat more warming foods and beverages, while in summer your body will crave cooling foods and refreshing beverages.

What puts many people off healthy eating habits is that nutritional advice keeps on changing and is often contradictory - one year we are told to avoid fats, and the next one to avoid carbohydrates. As nutritional science evolves, so does our understanding of what is healthy or not. However, catching up with the latest scientific results can be very confusing and exhausting.

On top of that, some diets include (or even insist on) expensive supplements, which may not be available everywhere, or which many people simply cannot afford. This is another reason why people are put off dieting.

The bottom line is, healthy eating habits should not be the prerogative of the rich, nor do they need to be complicated, expensive and boring. On the contrary.

Healthiest food is often the one which has been processed the least and which is as close to the way nature has made it as possible. Besides, for several different reasons- ranging from environmental, esoteric, and holistic - and Dr. Gundry's own research confirms this - it's best to eat local food and fruit and vegetable that are in season.

Basic Healthy Eating Guidelines - Regardless Of The Diet You May Be On

Adopt a healthy diet

There are many ways to eat healthily, so go for a diet which supports your lifestyle, and which consists of ingredients available locally.

Eat in tune with the seasons

Choosing seasonal and locally produced food is the easiest way to ensure you eat fresh and naturally ripened fruit and vegetable.

Eat slowly and chew food thoroughly

Studies show that food eaten slowly and chewed properly is not only easier to digest but is less fattening.

Stop eating before you feel full

If you eat slowly, you'll find it easy to know when you've had enough. By the time you feel full, you've already over-eaten.

Learn healthy cooking methods

As a rule of thumb, stir-fried and steamed vegetables are the healthiest way to cook. This way of cooking is also very convenient because it's easy and quick.

Enjoy your food

Never eat something you don't like. Food which you, for whatever reason, find disgusting, isn't nourishing. Your body is smart and knows what's best for you. There is a reason it reacts like that to certain foods - rather than force yourself to eat something just because it's supposed to be good for you, learn to listen to the subtle signs your body sends.

Stop obsessing about nutritional of each meal

This kill both the joy of cooking, as well as the joy of eating. Instead, learn to recognize the quality of food the way Orientals do: learn how certain foods affect your metabolism or your *dosha*.

Healthy doesn't have to mean tasteless

Find ways to bring even simple meals to life. With so many different kinds of natural spice to choose from, even a very restrictive diet's taste and appearance can be improved with a little bit of imagination. Learn to cook creatively.

Have your main meal before 6:00 PM

It would be best to have your main meal around noon because that's when your digestive fire is strongest.

Stop feeling guilty

Allow yourself to eat according to the 80/20 principle: eating healthy 80% of the time and treating yourself occasionally to something unhealthy (i.e. chocolate, pizza, etc.).

Healthy snacks

If you like eating between meals, always keep some fresh fruit or packs of dried fruit, nuts and seeds in your car, desk or bag).

Water, water, water!

Don't forget to drink water throughout the day. Drink at least 2 liters per day. In the winter drink only warm water or herbal teas.

Eat low-density food first

These are fresh fruit or vegetable which take up a lot of space in your stomach because they contain lots of fiber. This way, they make you feel full, even before you've started the meal. This is an easy way to trick yourself into eating less and eating healthy.

Don't keep unhealthy food at home.

It may be too tempting at times.

As Ann Wigmore, the American holistic health practitioner pointed out, "The food you eat can be either the safest and most powerful form of medicine or the slowest form of poison."

Food Energetics: The Power of Your Food Choices

The attitude to food, i.e., to the way it's prepared, served and eaten, differs fundamentally between the West and the East. The attention to detail, and an almost reverence-like attitude given to food in Asia, is in stark contrast to the way food is regarded and treated in the West. While Western cultures approach food in terms of calories, fat and protein content, in the East the food (and life in general) is seen in terms of energy and vibration.

In Asia, everything revolves around the idea of balance, and this is also the leading principle used when preparing food. One eats food suited to their constitution type (according to Ayurveda principles), or meals are prepared in accordance with the way they should affect your metabolism: to slow it down, warm it, cool it, dry it, etc. (according to the TCM principles).

What's behind the diametrically opposed approach to food of Western and Eastern cultures, is the worldview. In the materialistically oriented West, food is treated simply as a source of "fuel" which provides energy. In the East, where food is regarded as a source of *qi*, or life force which drives the world, food is taken seriously and is treated with respect. Besides, in the East, food is used as much for nutrition, as for healing. In other words, Eastern cultures view food holistically.

While in the West, we live fast, prepare fast meals and eat fast foods, in the East, enjoyment of meals is enhanced by relaxed, slow eating which also helps digestion. According to both Ayurveda and TCM, optimal health is the result of a healthy gut, and poor digestion is at the root of almost all health problems.

For the food to be digested properly, it needs to be cooked, served and eaten in a manner that facilitates digestion, which in turn, will facilitate absorption of nutrients.

On the other hand, in the West, we live in an increasingly stressful world where we are often forced to eat on the go, prepare meals in fast, unhealthy ways and when we shop we are often (mis)guided by aggressive advertising campaigns which are usually business-driven.

Besides, in the West, food is analyzed and broken down to atoms, in the hope it will help us understand nutrition principles better. In reality, it often confuses us even more because there are holistic aspects of food which cannot be explained by scientifically.

So, instead of spending endless time over-analyzing food components and trying to work out the amount of minerals, fats or protein you should take every day, try to enjoy your meals with all your senses: sight, smell, taste, and touch. For hygienic reasons, it's not always possible to eat with your hands (especially in public), but at least when you are at home discard the knife and fork and eat your food the way it was eaten for thousands of years – with your hands. Trust me, food eaten without cutlery, tastes different.

In case you wonder if it's possible to eat a Western diet and live in a Western culture and eat "Orientally", just by approaching your meals holistically, you can make a fundamental change in your attitude to food.

However, be warned. Adopting a holistic attitude to food in a culture obsessed with money, work, and appearance, where obesity and depression are getting epidemic proportions, is not easy.

As long as the food industry is allowed to spend millions of dollars on marketing usually very unhealthy foods, and as long as the aggressive advertising campaigns encourage eating fast foods, only those with a strong character will manage to turn the leaf.

7 simple steps to help you adopt "Oriental" eating habits:

Enjoy your food

Don't allow anyone to persuade you to eat something you don't like, just because it's supposed to be good for you. A recent Russian study revealed that if you eat something you can't stand (but still eat it because it's healthy, or because parents force you to eat it), such food becomes toxic once inside your body.

Besides, never underestimate the importance of joy in your life. Just like psychologists claim that enjoying what you do for a living (or getting involved in a hobby you enjoy) has a major influence on your mental health, so the food eaten with joy and appetite is more nourishing and less fattening because metabolism works better with food you eat with pleasure.

Make yourself comfortable during meals

Whenever possible, try to eat at a table, in a comfortable chair, and in a relaxed atmosphere. Don't read while you eat or listen to the news. Try not to talk too much during meals, and if feeling upset, angry or anxious, it's best to postpone the meal until you have calmed down.

Eating while you are in "a state" can make you eat emotionally and this usually means you will eat comfort food (i.e. junk food), or you will overeat, or you will give yourself stomach cramps later. When we are upset or angry our stomach tends to get "tied in a knot" which makes digestion almost impossible. Besides, we don't focus on food because we are thinking about the issues that made us angry or anxious. Such meals usually end up with indigestion, bloating or even vomiting.

Chew well and eat slowly

Food chewed thoroughly is already half-digested by the time it reaches the stomach, and this helps digestion. Besides, when you eat slowly you usually eat less because you start feeling full in time to stop before you've overeaten.

Avoid too much liquid during, and immediately after meals

Water should be taken 30 minutes before, and 2 hours after the meal. If you have to drink something during the meal, make sure it's never more than a small cup of warm water or tea.

Avoid eating cold foods, even in summer

Your stomach needs "fire" to digest your meal and cold foods tend to dampen and weaken this fire. Raw salads are good if the main meal is warm. Asian meals are made from warming (yang) foods during cold months, or are prepared in a way that gives them more yang qualities. Equally, during hot summer months, Chinese cooking focuses on yin foods or cooking methods which make food yin (i.e. cooling). But, regardless of the season, the most important factor of both Ayurveda and TCM cooking is maintaining the balance.

Know when to stop

If you think you will struggle to stop before you feel full, fill your plate with the amount of food you think you should eat to stop yourself from taking a second helping. If you can, rest for half an hour after a meal, as this helps digestion

Eat local and organic food whenever possible

Locally produced food is best for you. Of course, this is not always possible, but if you have a choice, always go for local.

Food for Thought: Mindfulness and Food Absorption

Living, and eating, mindfully is about "being present". Too often, we just rush through a day (or life) without ever finding the time to stop and notice where we're going (or think about what we're eating).

When it comes to food, we often eat at our desk while reading e-mails, while queuing at the bus stop, or while driving to work in the morning. Food gulped down mindlessly isn't nourishing. At best, it's simply "fuel" so you can carry on.

We are not machines and the food we eat should be more than just a source of energy. We are spiritual beings and the food should also satisfy our emotional and spiritual needs. Eating mindfully is about learning to appreciate the flavors, colors or ingredients of your meal.

5 ways of introducing mindfulness into your eating habits:

Listen to your body

Why do we so often ignore the signals our body sends trying to tell us something is wrong? Constant headaches warn of a stressful life and mean we should slow down. Poor digestion is a warning our diet is wrong. Cravings for certain foods often mean that certain nutrients are missing in our diet. Try to tune in with your body and learn to hear and recognize the signals it sends you.

Show respect

Food is the essence of life and it deserves to be treated with respect. When you compare how food is selected, prepared, served and eaten in some cultures, the way the Western countries treat food is atrocious. Even if you ignore the fact that thousands of tons of food are wasted every year in developed countries, the processed food which is the basis of our diet, is produced and prepared in a way that usually destroys all the nutrients. Food deserves better treatment.

There is a reason people used to say grace before each meal. To change your attitude to food and learn the art of mindful eating, start paying attention to the food that supports your life. You don't have to say grace, but feeling grateful for having food to eat, is already a step to mindful living. Stop wasting food, buy only what you need, prepare your meals with minimal cooking and eat it when you feel calm.

Preparing food mindfully

As you prepare the food, notice how it looks, smells and feels under your fingers. Notice the color changing as you cook it, notice how taste improves as you add spice. I read about a woman who said that the only time she could find for herself in her busy life, was when she was making bread. She enjoyed this ME time so much, she turned it into a weekly meditation practice. As she mixed the flour and spices, kneaded the dough, waited for it to rise, and then enjoyed the smell of freshly baked bread, she was transported from her stressful and hectic world into a different dimension.

Preparing food mindfully, whether it's baking a cake, preparing a salad or making a curry, helps you switch off from the mundane concerns and worries. Enjoy the cooking process (if you can) and regard this time as a transition time, during which you relax and "switch off", so you feel calm and "centered" by the time the meal is ready.

Saying grace before a meal has the same purpose. In those couple of minutes, you stop all your thoughts and focus on something else. You don't even have to say grace, just sit quietly for a moment, relaxing, winding down and changing your focus from everyday problems to food.

Eat focused on what's on your plate

Eating slowly not only improves your digestion, it also helps the food nutrients be absorbed more efficiently, making the food not only more nourishing but also less fattening. Try to ignore noises that can catch your attention, and rather focus on the different flavors, shapes, and colors in your plate.

Although many of these tips are difficult to stick to in our frantically busy world, adopting one of these tips at a time will help you change your attitude to food and to the food-related activities, such as shopping, preparing, cooking, serving, eating. As your pleasure for food grows, so will your eagerness to adopt a more mindful lifestyle.

As the British-Canadian novelist, Elizabeth Thornton put it, "Mindfulness is a way of being present: paying attention to and accepting what is happening in our lives. It helps us to be aware of, and step away from our automatic and habitual reactions to our everyday experiences".

Eating automatically and habitually is the way you eat while watching TV. On the other hand, eating mindfully is about stepping out of your comfort zone when it comes to food – treating it respectfully, preparing it lovingly and consuming it with joy.

Chapter 2

What Makes Healthy Food Unhealthy?

There are many ways to destroy your health, and one of the easiest ones is with unhealthy food choices.

A typical Western diet revolves around processed food, which is why the surge of diet-related diseases is not surprising. We now know that the so-called diseases of civilization (cancer, stroke, heart disease, autoimmune disease, obesity, diabetes), are directly linked to a diet rich in saturated fats and sugars, and sedentary lifestyle.

Unfortunately, junk food is usually very tasty, thanks to a large amount of flavor and color additives, salt, fats, and sugar. Besides, although it has very little, or no nutritional value, it's very convenient, as most of it is prepackaged and ready to use, e.g. frozen meals, processed meats, sweets, breads, etc.

On the other hand, natural foods, i.e. fruit, vegetable, whole grains and good fats, are not only nutritious, they even have the power to help you reverse effects of many life-threatening diseases, as shown in the *China Study* by Dr. Colin Campbell.

However, the increasingly toxic environment affects the quality and safety even of healthy foods. Therefore, eliminating, or at least reducing environmental toxins from your diet should be your main priority, for although there may be nothing you can do about global warming, there are ways of preventing toxins from getting into your body through food.

Another thing to bear in mind is that choosing natural, healthy foods, but then preparing them in a way that destroys most of their nutrients, or makes them difficult to be absorbed or digested, is as bad as eating junk food.

As Michael Pollan, an American professor and natural food activities wrote in one of his books, "There are a great many food-like items in the supermarket your ancestors wouldn't recognize as food...stay away from these."

The first step on your path to wellness is including healthy foods in your diet. The next one should be learning how to preserve their nutrients and enable your body to benefit from them.

Anti-Nutrients

Most of us have heard about the potentially very negative effects of the so-called anti-nutrients on our health.

Anti-nutrients are chemical compounds found in plants which serve as a defense mechanism against predators (including humans). These compounds help repel various pests until the fruit is ripe and ready to be eaten. By making the unripe fruit and vegetable-rich with lectins (and thus unpleasant and unhealthy for consumption), a plant ensures its fruit is protected until the seeds are ready to germinate.

Anti-nutrients are particularly prominent in grains, beans, legumes, and nuts. They are also found in most fruit and vegetables, but in much smaller quantities.

The main problem with anti-nutrients is that they interfere with absorption of vitamins and minerals. Ideally, we should avoid them, but as they are found in almost all foods, this may not be possible for practical reasons. Besides, some of the anti-nutrient rich foods are very nutritious, so removing them from your diet could do more harm than good.

5 most common anti-nutrients:

Lectins

Lectins are found in high quantities in grains and legumes. They are believed to be the main cause of indigestion, bloating and gas. Since many of them survive digestion by the gastrointestinal tract, they easily penetrate cells lining.

When that happens, lectins can wreak havoc on your digestive tract by interfering with nutrient absorption, disrupting the gut flora, slowing down digestion and even triggering autoimmune reactions. Inadequately prepared grains, dairy and legumes like peanuts, and soybeans are particularly unhealthy.

Gluten

Found in wheat, rye, and barley, this protein is particularly difficult to digest and is well-known for causing many gastrointestinal problems and allergies. Besides, it can contribute to the leaky gut syndrome and some autoimmune diseases.

Being gluten intolerant means giving up all the foods that contain it, which is what we usually eat a lot of: breads, pastas, cereals, crackers, etc. The trouble is that even grains that don't contain a lot of gluten, such as oats, quinoa, rice or corn, easily become contaminated during the storing, production or packaging process, if these take place in a facility used for wheat processing.

Besides, gluten is found in many food additives, which means that many foods which we believe to be gluten-free, contain gluten, e.g. salad dressings, salami, sweets, etc. For this reason, giving up gluten completely is practically impossible.

Phytic Acid

This is probably the best-known anti-nutrient and is found in grains, beans, nuts, and potatoes. It binds to minerals and prevents their absorption, sometimes leading to deficiencies, especially if your diet is high in fiber and whole-grain foods.

However, phytates are also an antioxidant and help fight some cancers. The best way to benefit from them without causing yourself too much harm, is to balance the amount of high-phytate foods you include in your diet, while getting enough of the nutrients that phytate destroys, from supplements.

Saponins

Similar to lectins, saponins affect the gastrointestinal lining, contributing to the leaky gut syndrome and autoimmune disorders. They're particularly resistant to digestion and can enter the bloodstream and trigger immune responses.

Saponins occur naturally in soybeans, peas, ginseng, herbs, vegetables, and yucca. They are used in beverages, as well as in cosmetics.

Solanine

Found in eggplant, peppers, and tomatoes, this is a very healthy anti-nutrient, unless consumed in high doses, particularly if you are sensitive to eating nightshades. An overdose of solanine can cause symptoms like those of real poisoning such as nausea, diarrhea, vomiting, stomach cramps, burning of the throat, headaches, and dizziness.

Avoiding anti-nutrients is both difficult (because they are found almost in all foods), and potentially harmful (because some of them are actually very healthy), so the best way to address the potential side-effects is to reduce the amount of food that contains anti-nutrients in your diet.

Easy ways of reducing the amount of anti-nutrients:

Replace anti-nutrient-rich foods with alternative foods

For example, you can use millet and tapioca instead of wheat.

Lower the content of anti-nutrients in anti-nutrient rich foods

Soaking, sprouting and fermenting significantly reduces the content of anti-nutrients in certain foods.

Soaking rice and beans for 24 hours, then cooking them for the longest time possible, can reduce some anti-nutrients by 50%.

Fermentation is an ancient way of preparing and preserving food. During this natural process, microorganisms such as bacteria or yeasts, start digesting carbs in food. This process is used when preparing wine, beer, cheese, yogurt, coffee, cocoa, sauerkraut.

Boiling

One study showed that boiling, especially at high heat, can reduce up to 70% of lectin and tannin.

Combination methods

Experiments show that anti-nutrients react differently to various food preparation methods and that the most effective way to reduce them in plant foods is to combine several different elimination strategies. That way they are destroyed almost completely.

Some people are more sensitive to anti-nutrients than others, so if you know that a particular food contains a lot of anti-nutrients, eat it only occasionally, or in small quantities.

Environmental toxins

It's no secret that chemically treated crops have a different nutritional quality compared to those produced organically. Besides, modern farming methods not only poison the crops by chemical fertilizers but in the long term, they also deplete the soil of basic nutrients.

Although this is an on-going debate, laboratory tests show that organically-grown fruits and vegetables have significantly more anti-oxidants, polyphenols, and enzymes. Unfortunately, as most of us eat commercially produced food, this means that our health is being slowly, but steadily undermined and destroyed by the food which is both chemically contaminated, and low in nutrients.

Another reason (and it brings us back to the problems of anti-nutrients), behind our nutritional deficiencies, is that fruits and vegetables are now being picked before they are ripe. To make them more appealing and immediately available for sale, many fruits and vegetables are treated chemically to make them look ripe. The best example is tomato.

The trouble is that fruits and vegetables picked up before they are ripe, contain more lectin than they would have if allowed to ripen naturally. The reason for this is that the mother plant is trying to protect its "child" from being eaten before the seeds are ready to germinate and produce new life the following year. The plant protects its fruit by making sure it contains a high dose of lectins which will make the predator sick.

To extend their shelf life, most fruits and vegetables, especially the imported ones, are picked well before they are ripe, which means that most of them contain much more lectin than is good for us.

The food we eat today is nutritionally very different from the food available 50 years ago. Most of our food is chemically "infested" to a certain degree.

Toxins present in water, soil, and air, will sooner or later be absorbed by plants that will pass them on to us once they become part of our diet. The buildup of environmental toxins is a common cause of health problems.

Plants absorb pollutants in three ways:

Water

Most of the water bodies, especially those near urban areas, are highly polluted. Main pollutants are pesticides and fertilizers from crop fields, animal waste from farms and garbage and dangerous chemicals dumped legally or illegally by individuals or industries. Heavily polluted water usually kills plants, but it is also absorbed by the plant root system and later enters our own system when such a plant becomes part of your diet.

Soil

Soil becomes polluted from runoffs or polluted water. Some of the highly carcinogenic contaminants commonly found in soil are found in certain dyes, plastics, and pesticides and have been linked to low birth weight, premature delivery, heart malformations, lower IQ and childhood asthma. In adults, long exposure to foods from such soils can cause damage to their lungs, kidney, liver, and skin.

Air

Most of the air pollution comes from car exhaust fumes and industry. Heavy air pollution kills plants or makes them very unhealthy, especially if they are located near busy roads, which many agricultural fields are. Lead is particularly prominent in such fruit, vegetable, and honey.

Protecting yourself and your food from the major sources of environmental toxins is becoming a full-time job. Crops absorb toxins from the soil, water, and air and once consumed as food, traces of those toxins can be found in your body. Our liver works nonstop to rid us of toxins, but if they reach a level it can no longer process, our body starts storing them.

2 ways of avoiding toxins in food:

1. Avoid toxic foods
2. Detox yourself from accumulated toxins

You can avoid, or significantly reduce the amount of toxins in your food (and your body) by buying organic foods, and by drinking and cooking with filtered water. However, if this is not possible, at least be aware of some facts:

- Certain fruits and vegetables are chemically treated once a week from the moment they bloom until they are picked (a period of about 3 months) and are therefore considered extremely toxic. Among such food are peaches, apples, bell peppers, strawberries, cherries, imported grapes, spinach, lettuce, potato.
- Farmed or Atlantic salmon should also be avoided. It is naturally white and to make it resemble wild salmon, it is fed pellets that contain pink dye. Farmed salmon is fed mainly groundfish and soy. Besides, to further cut the production costs, many salmon farmers add poultry poop and chicken feathers to the food. (NOTE: Alaskan salmon is safe to eat).
- Fish with high mercury content: shark, swordfish, tuna, king mackerel, marlin, halibut, snapper is unfortunately now considered extremely unhealthy, due to the dumping of millions of tons

of mercury into the seas and oceans. (NOTE: fish with lower mercury content which is safe to eat is sardines, clam, ocean perch, sole, catfish).

You can significantly reduce the amount of toxins in your body if you avoid these foods, but you can also reduce your toxic load by introducing certain foods in your diet.

Most helpful detox foods:

- Leafy greens. The darker the green color, the higher the chlorophyll content and the more toxins it will help destroy.
- Two to three cups of green tea per day will ensure your body stores sufficient quantity of antioxidants to boost your immune system.
- To deal with unhealthy chemicals in fruit and vegetables, get into the habit of soaking them in a mixture of equal quantities of water, vinegar (or lemon juice) and bicarbonate of soda for 20 minutes.

Unhealthy Cooking and Food Preservation Methods

There's no point in buying natural foods if you are going to destroy them by unhealthy cooking methods. Even organically produced food becomes worthless if cooked in a way that destroys its nutrients, color or flavor.

Choosing healthy food is important, but the way the food is cooked also counts. Healthy cooking methods principle is about changing the food as little as possible from its natural appearance and preserving as much of its color, flavor, and nutrients.

The usual methods of cooking involve boiling, grilling, frying, stewing, deep-frying, and most of them are very unhealthy. This is partly because long cooking time destroys the nutrients, and partly because such food becomes full of saturated fats.

3 most unhealthy cooking methods:

Deep-frying

This is cooking in deep, hot oil and is one of the unhealthiest ways to cook. It increases the saturated fat content of the food and is the major reason for weight gain and high cholesterol levels.

Charcoal grilling (Barbecue)

Some consider grilling a healthy way of preparing food (particularly meat) because no additional fats are used in cooking. However, charcoal grilled food is linked to increased risk of cancer. The solution might be to replace the charcoal barbecue with an electrical one.

Boiling

Boiling food for too long, or in too much water, or with the open lid, will affect the nutritional quality of the meal since most of the nutrients are destroyed in prolonged cooking or are absorbed by water. Water steals the nutrients from the food cooked in it, which is why broths are so healing – all the nutrients from the meat or vegetable have been extracted by the water. However, if you use only vegetables or meat and throw away the water they were cooked in, you lose a considerable amount of nutrients. Besides, cooking in very high heat destroys about 20% of some vitamins - especially vitamin C.

On the other hand, some studies suggest that certain foods benefit from cooking. When cooking carrots, spinach, and tomatoes, for example, heat facilitates the release of antioxidants by breaking down cell walls, making it easier for our digestive tract to absorb the nutrients these vegetables are full of.

3 healthy cooking methods:

Steaming

Cooking food in its own juice is considered the healthiest way of food preparation.

Stir-frying

Used mainly in Chinese cooking, it greatly improves flavor because the food absorbs only a little bit of oil, as it's cooked in just a few minutes. However, for the cooking process to be short and healthy, food needs to be chopped up into small pieces.

Boiling lightly

If boiling is your favorite way of cooking, you can improve the nutritional value of food cooked this way by cooking it in as little water as possible, with the lid on and over moderate heat.

Another important element of cooking is food preservation. Various preservation methods have been used for millennia, especially in cold parts of the world where the growing season is short. Your diet can be greatly improved if you master the techniques which will enable you to have access to otherwise unavailable fruit and vegetable throughout the year.

6 most common methods of food preservation are:

Fermentation

This method of food preservation has been used for thousands of years because it allows foods to stay edible longer. Lacto-fermentation enhances the nutritive value of the food, and many enzymes and probiotics are created in the process. It involves chopping up vegetables, mixing them with some salt and water, and allowing them to ferment.

Acidification

Many foods last longer if they are soaked in vinegar, the most common ones being cucumbers, beets, carrots, and peppers. This is an ancient method of food preservation, and different acids can be used.

Canning

Proper canning techniques prevent food spoilage by exposing it to heat. Canning also requires that air is removed from jars and a vacuum formed as the jars cool and seal. This is the way jams, tomatoes, chutneys, and condiments are preserved.

Drying

Fruit, vegetable, meat, and fish can be dried in different ways. Sun drying takes 3-4 days and requires very hot and dry air conditions (suitable for fruit). Air drying takes place indoors in a well-ventilated attic or room (suitable for herbs and hot peppers). Dehydrators ensure all the ingredients have been dried uniformly and hygienically. Microwave drying is a quick way of drying small quantities of herbs and leaf vegetables (2-3 minutes).

Smoking

Since smoke is antimicrobial and antioxidant it is used to preserve foods. Smoking is probably the oldest food preservation method and could have developed shortly after fire was discovered. The most common smoked foods are meat and fish, although there are many other foods which are improved with smoke flavor, e.g. cheese, nuts, vegetables, whiskey, etc.

Freezing

A healthy way of preserving fresh fruit and vegetables, although you need to have a reliable source of electricity.

PART 2

Chapter 3

Plant Paradox Eating Habits

Making the switch

Deciding to change your diet is one thing but sticking to it is quite another. It's well-known that the reason most diets fail is that they are unsustainable in the long term. You follow the directions, you achieve what you were told you would achieve (i.e. you lose weight, or your cholesterol level improves, or your blood pressure drops, etc.), but the moment you go back to your old diet, the weight, and cholesterol return. The reason for this is that many popular diets are impractical, or difficult to follow over a long period of time, so you sooner or later have to go back to how you used to eat.

Some diets are difficult to follow, some require expensive supplements or food items unavailable to everyone, some require eating routines that are incompatible with a busy lifestyle. But, what is probably the biggest reason people find it difficult to adopt a new eating habit, are their current eating habits.

I read somewhere that diet is as important as culture and is just as difficult to change permanently. But, if you've made up your mind about changing your diet, do it slowly and have a plan. Set a goal and a timeframe within which you hope to achieve some results (e.g. lose a certain amount of weight, or switch to a completely different eating plan).

If this is going to be a major change (e.g. like switching from an omnivore to a vegan, or if you want to detox by living only on water and juices for 6 weeks), you will have to think this through and be aware of possible side-effects. Besides, it's crucial you make sure you have no health issues which could be made worse by a drastic diet change.

If you think you'll struggle adopting the Plant Paradox diet, start by changing your diet slowly, gradually introducing more and more vegetables, into your meals, while reducing the amount of grains, dairy, and meat. That way, on the day you decide to start preparing your body for the Plant Paradox diet, the change will not drastic.

One of the ways of adopting a different diet or introducing healthy eating habits, is to "trick" your body into eating healthy foods without having to give up on the foods it's used to. This is called "crowding out" and it works like this:

Instead of giving up on unhealthy foods, you simply add healthy foods to your diet. It works best when you eat the healthy food first, and then allow yourself to have the less-healthy food later (i.e. when you're already full).

However, whenever considering a diet change, especially a drastic one, it helps to consider some other factors. For example, if you are planning cutting down on calories and carbohydrates, it's probably better to do this in summer, because cold winter months will make it more difficult to feel full on decreased calories.

If you want to go on a detox diet which requires living on fresh juice for six weeks, it makes sense to do it in the season when such produce is available, rather than using frozen fruit and veg.

Dr. Gundry's advice for switching to Plant Paradox diet is to first prepare your body for the changes that will occur in it once you stop consuming lectins. What you must be aware of is that if you've been eating lactin- and sugar-rich foods for a long time, your gut is probably full of bad bacteria, that will sabotage your attempts to switch to healthy eating, by constant cravings the unhealthy foods.

The good news is that when you change your diet, your gut can benefit immediately. All you need to do to ensure a smooth transition is prepare your body properly, so it doesn't experience the new diet as a shock. In case you wonder what you need to do to repair the damage that years of unhealthy eating habits have done to your gut, it's simple - all you need to do is remove lectins from your diet.

According to Dr. Gundry, you shouldn't eat these foods during the three-day preparation period:

- Dairy
- Grains
- Fruit
- Sugar
- Seeds
- Eggs
- Soy
- Nightshade plants
- Roots
- Tubers
- Corn
- Soy
- Certain oils
- Farm animal proteins

Foods you <u>should</u> eat during the three-day preparation period:

Basically, these are cruciferous vegetables and leafy greens. The choice is big, so regardless of where you live or what the season is, you will have lots of healthy vegetables to choose from. You can eat as much as you want to, either cooked or raw. Whenever possible, try to eat organic.

- Broccoli
- Brussels sprouts
- Cauliflower
- Bok choy
- Cabbage
- Chinese cabbage
- Swiss chard
- Arugula
- Watercress
- Collards
- Kale
- Radicchio
- Raw sauerkraut
- Kimchi
- Nopales cactus
- Celery
- Onions
- Leeks
- Chives
- Scallions
- Chicory
- Carrots
- Carrot greens
- Artichokes

- Beets
- Radishes
- Daikon radishes
- Hearts of palm
- Cilantro
- Okra
- Asparagus
- Garlic
- Romaine
- Leafy greens
- Kohlrabi
- Mesclun
- Spinach
- Endive
- Dandelion greens
- Butter lettuce
- Fennel
- Escarole
- Mustard greens
- Mizuna
- Parsley
- Basil
- Mint
- Purslane
- Perilla
- Algae
- Seaweed
- Sea vegetables
- Mushrooms

Other allowed foods:

<u>Protein</u>: You can eat fish or pastured chicken, but not more than 200 gr per day.

<u>Oils</u>: Use only good oils, and avoid all those not on this list:

- Avocado oil
- Coconut oil
- Macadamia nut oil
- Sesame seed oil
- Walnut oil
- Extra-virgin olive oil
- Hemp seed oil
- Flaxseed oil

<u>Dressing</u>: Fresh, home-made ones are best. The easiest, and probably the healthiest one, is olive oil and lemon juice. But, you can also use vinegar, mustard, black pepper, sea salt, fresh herbs and fresh spices.

<u>Drink</u>: Water, or unsweetened tea.

Depending on how unhealthy your life has been, your body may find it difficult to adjust to healthy eating habits in just three days. Don't force a new diet upon yourself. If you are struggling, introduce changes slowly, even if it means extending the prep period to a week, or longer. Once your body accepts the change, it will be easy to switch to the Plant Paradox diet.

Plants Can Heal, Plants Can Kill

Without plants, there would be no life on earth. They provide food, heating, building material, housing, and of course, food for ourselves and all the herbivores we feed on. But, although we regard plants mainly as a source of food, we often forget they can also be medicine.

2 ways plants can cure and heal:

As part of a healthy diet

This was recognized thousands of years ago in India and China, where food is used both as nourishment and for healing (physical, mental, and spiritual).

As medicine

There is plenty of archaeological and written evidence that plants were used for healing since prehistoric times. Even today, when feeling unwell, many people first turn to nature for help. They seek relief in clay, leeches, herbs, plants, healing springs, clean mountain air, etc.

Plant-Based Diets and Your Health

A plant-based diet is one of the best ways to eat. Even those who promote non-vegetarian, or purely animal-protein diets (e.g. Paleo), stress the importance of eating fresh fruit and vegetable as much as possible. In other words, everyone agrees that fruits and vegetables are crucial for a healthy diet.

7 reasons plants are vital for your health:

- They are a rich source of vitamins and minerals
- Some plants are a rich source of protein
- Plant-based diet is easy to digest
- Fresh fruit and vegetable is known to have revitalizing and rejuvenating properties
- Juicing is part of almost all detox methods
- Plant production causes less environmental degradation

- Plant-based diet promotes longevity and prevents many diseases

However, even healthy plants under certain conditions can become unhealthy.

5 most common ways of making healthy food unhealthy:

Wrong cooking methods

Deep frying, cooking in too much water, using too much flavor and color additives, etc.

Wrong storing methods

Exposing food to light and heat destroys it within days or hours.

Wrong preservation methods

Using too many chemical additives can make food not only unhealthy but downright toxic.

Wrong food combining

Certain food combinations or practices can wreak havoc on your health: eating fruit immediately after a meal, cheese and meat omelet, tomato and cheese pasta sauce, banana and milk, yogurt with fruit, lemon dressing with tomato or cucumber salad, etc.

Wrong time for eating

Eating late at night, or when stressed, or when in a rush, is guaranteed to give you indigestion. Food stays in the gut for too long, begins to rot.

On the other hand, certain healthy plant-based foods can cause serious health problems:

Allergies

As food allergies continue to rise, doctors struggle to understand how come about 90% of allergic reactions come from these eight foods alone: milk, eggs, peanuts, tree nuts, soy, wheat, fish, and shellfish. Although many aspects of our modern lives are working together to make allergies more common, it's obvious that it's the dairy and lectin-rich foods which are the main allergens. Besides, climate change and rising carbon dioxide levels increase the amount of pollen in the air, and the ability of that pollen to cause allergies.

Indigestible foods

Lectin-rich foods contribute, and may even cause, many autoimmune diseases and digestive disorders, including leaky gut.

Headaches

Red wine and chocolate often act as headache triggers. Wine, because of the sulfites used as preservatives, and chocolate, due to the two chemicals it contains: tyramine and phenylalanine.

Plant Medicine

Modern medicine has accepted many of the traditional healing methods, often finding out about them by accident. A typical example of this is how the well-known cardiotonic was discovered by a physician who persistently failed to bring about improvement in a patient suffering from severe dropsy caused by heart failure. Suddenly, the patient started to recover. His relatives admitted giving him an herbal tea of foxglove based on an old family recipe. Further research proved this plant to be very therapeutic, and it's still used today to produce *digitoxin*, a well-known cardiotonic for heart-related problems.

List of medicine made from plants is very long because there are over a hundred active ingredients derived from plants for use as drugs and medicines. These are some of them:

- Aescin, an <u>anti-inflammatory</u> medicine made from horse chestnut
- Berberine, treatment for bacillary <u>dysentery</u>, made from common barberry
- Betulinic acid, <u>anti-cancerous</u> drug, made from common birch
- Cocaine, local <u>anesthetic</u>, made from coca plant
- Colchiceine amide, <u>anti-tumor</u> drug, made from autumn crocus
- Kawain, <u>tranquilizer</u>, made from kava kava
- Santonin, <u>ascaricid</u>, made from wormwood
- Thymol, <u>anti-fungal</u>, made from thyme
- Vasicine, <u>cerebral stimulant</u>, made from periwinkle

However, besides the ability to heal, many plants contain ingredients that can cause harm. And it's not just the matter of eating poisonous mushrooms or plants, it's more often the case of overdosing, or using the wrong part of the plant.

Fresh fruit and vegetables are crucial for a healthy diet, but some parts of some fruit and vegetable (mainly the stone and skin), contain small amounts of natural toxins which can cause digestive problems if consumed in large quantities, or by someone with a particularly sensitive digestive system.

A typical example is kernels of apricots, cherries, peaches, and prunes. They are powerful herbal supplements for both skin care and diet and are known to be very nutritious, but only if consumed in small quantities.

Apricot

The kernels of apricots, cherries, peaches, pears, plums, and prunes contain a chemical which when chewed, transforms into cyanide. Although the flesh doesn't contain any toxin, kernels do and should be eaten only in small quantities, i.e. not more than five per day, particularly if you eat then on the regular basis.

Almonds

Almonds are one of the healthiest nuts, even though they are full of cyanide. However, there's no need to worry, for the poison is found mainly in bitter, or wild almonds and these contain about 50 times more cyanide than sweet almonds, which is the kind available in shops. The poison is removed by thermal processing, e.g. y-irradiation, dry roasting, blanching, oil roasting and other methods.

Cherries

Cherries are a very popular fruit – used in cooking, liqueur production, or eaten raw. Besides, they are not only tasty, but are packed with vitamins and minerals, and antioxidants. Sweet cherries are particularly healthy, especially the dark red ones. The darker the skin, the more antioxidants they contain. However, the stones of cherries contain a type of hydrogen cyanide, and although crushed cherry stones are added to liquors to improve the flavor, try not to chew on the pip for too long, especially if it's crushed.

Potatoes

Potatoes produce certain chemicals which, in small doses, improve the flavor of cooked potatoes, but if consumed in large doses, they induce poison-like symptoms. Unfortunately, these chemicals, glycoalkaloids, are not destroyed by heat, so cooking or frying won't help you get rid of it. Fortunately, most of this chemical is found in the skin, or just below, so removing the skin before cooking, baking or frying, solves the problem. To last, potatoes should be stored in dark, cool place, and you should always avoid those which are beginning to sprout or go green. Potato poisoning is very rare and can be avoided by proper storing, as well as preparation and cooking methods.

Carrots

Unusual flavor of carrots may mean that they were intentionally, or unintentionally exposed to a fruit ripening hormone, ethylene. To avoid this kind of contamination, it's best not to store carrots with fruit and vegetable for which the ripening hormone is regularly used, such as apples, avocados, bananas, peaches, tomatoes, etc.

Elderberry

Elderberry trees are used mainly for their delicate flowers (from which we make tea or liquor) and berries (which are used to make jams, juice or syrup). Leaves can also be used to make ointments, and bark as a liver stimulant, however, these are highly poisonous, as are the roots. Therefore, extreme care should be taken when picking the flower or the fruit, so as not to pick stems or leaves as well.

Castor oil

Castor oil is usually used for stomach troubles, but it is also added to many foods, such as candies and chocolate. Castor bean, from which the oil is made, is an extremely poisonous plant. Only one bean is sufficient to kill a human, so it needs to be carefully processed before it becomes safe to use as medication. Although in small quantities it heals, the poison *ricin* is very toxic and workers who harvest the plant need to be protected by masks and gloves.

Chapter 4

What's so Special About Plant Paradox Diet

Do you sometimes wish you could go back to eating habits like those before the grains and dairy became our staple diet, and live and eat as our ancestors did – in tune with the seasons? If you do, it's probably because you are one of the growing number of people who feel that the obesity, autoimmune diseases, and depression epidemic, has something to do with the modern diet.

Plant Paradox is an unorthodox, and somewhat controversial attempt to help us postpone aging and get rid of autoimmune diseases and digestive disorders brought on by a diet based on processed foods, grains and dairy. Although milk and whole grains were traditionally regarded as very healthy, modern farming methods have changed them so much during hundreds of years of hybridization and toxic food additives, that they are no longer considered safe to eat.

However, the real problem behind these health issues is not only the food. Our immune system was designed to resist most of the diseases. Unfortunately, decades of unhealthy diets, sedentary lifestyle, overuse of antibiotics and high-stress levels, have weakened and degraded our body's self-defense to such a level that today, most people seem to suffer from constant fatigue, insomnia, depression, recurrent infections or autoimmune diseases.

Plant Paradox is a revolutionary approach to eliminating many health problems by re-activating your immune response through a lectin-free diet. A revitalized and healthy body will not only be strong enough to tackle infections and inflammations but will help you age with dignity.

Key Principles

After curing himself of obesity and chronic disease with a change of diet, Dr. Steven Gundry, a cardiologist turned nutritionist, developed the Plant Paradox programme, focusing his research on the comparison of food quality today, with that of the pre-Neolithic times.

Scientific evidence confirms that hunter-gatherers consumed about 250 species of plants as part of their diet, and that the animals they hunted for food, consumed the same plants. The saying "You are what you eat", made Dr. Gundry think that there must be a link between the kind of food we eat and we feed the animals we eat with, and the state of our health, AND the food eaten by both people and animals in the pre-Neolithic times, and the state of their health. Many years of research made him realize that it was the difference in both variety and quality of plant food, that is behind the growing number of chronic diseases, especially in the developed world.

He came up with a dietary regime that not only helps with weight loss, but that can reverse and eradicate serious diseases, such as high blood pressure, and in some cases even cancer.

Years of research and experiments made it clear that most autoimmune diseases and digestive disorders could be cured with a lectin-free diet, but also that the same health problems would come back as soon as lectin was reintroduced into the diet.

The Plant Paradox regime helped thousands of people get rid of the "incurable" autoimmune diseases and various digestive problems, and the best part of it is, the philosophy behind the Plant Paradox is basically very simple. It revolves around four time-tested healthy-eating habits.

4 key principles of the Plant Paradox dietary regime are:

1. Remove lectins from your diet
2. Practice intermittent fasting
3. Eat according to the Plant Paradox Food Pyramid
4. Eat (and live) in tune with the seasons

Remove lectins from your diet

Lectins are plant proteins found in almost 30% of the food we eat but are particularly concentrated in grains and legumes. Fruits and vegetables also contain them but in smaller quantities.

Some lectins are toxic and inflammatory, and those with a lectin-intolerance can experience serious digestive problems after eating lectin-rich foods, such as bloating, gas, nausea, diarrhea, etc. Lectins are also believed to be partially responsible for creating a "leaky gut" that leads to autoimmune disease.

The trouble with lectins is that they are resistant to cooking and digestive enzymes, which means some of them manage to go through the gut wall unaltered and enter the blood. They can also damage the walls of the intestines by attaching to them and thickening them, which affects their nutrient absorption ability.

Although not all lectins are bad, some can be VERY bad. For example, castor beans (from which castor oil is made) contain so many lectins that they are poisonous to most animals. The lectin found in castor bean has even been synthesized as a poison called *ricin*, which is used in biochemical warfare.

There is a growing number of nutritionists who believe that 10,000 years that have passed since the agriculture revolution drastically changed our lifestyle and diet, was insufficient time for our digestive system to adapt to a diet dominated by grains, legumes, and dairy. The crux of the problem is that humans don't have the proper enzymes necessary to digest lectins and therefore react to them as "foreign".

Practice intermittent fasting

Many cultures and detox methods recommend regular, or occasional, fasting as a natural way of self-cleansing.

Plant Paradox theory advocates water fasting as a way of improving your metabolism and activating autophagy. Autophagy is derived from the Greek *auto* (self) and *phagein* (to eat). Literally translated, it means "self-eating".

Yorshinori Ohsumi, a Japanese cell biologist who received the 2016 Nobel Prize in Physiology for his discoveries of mechanisms for autophagy, described it as an activity which rids our body of old cells it no longer needs.

The key activator of autophagy is nutrient deprivation. So, basically, once you deprive your body of food, it starts fighting for survival. The first thing it does is identify old and sick cells and decides to get rid of them for they no longer serve any purpose. Seen from the point of self-detox, autophagy can also be regarded as a major regenerative process, during which your body cleanse and rejuvenates itself.

Not only is autophagy good for self-regeneration, it's also believed that the accumulation of old cells is one of the triggers of premature aging. Studies even show that some of the consequences of heavy accumulation of old cells and other cellular junk, are Alzheimer's disease and cancer.

In the pre-agriculture days, autophagy used to happen seasonally, as soon as winter set in. People generally ate irregularly, and during winter months, they sometimes went without food for days. Sometimes, they starved even during the summer months, due to flooding, drought, disease, etc. However, summer was usually the time during which they gorged on fruit, honey, meat, fish and anything else they could find. That way they stored enough fat for winter.

Abstaining from food, unless, of course, it goes on for too long, is believed to be the best natural way for the body to detox and repair itself.

According to Plant Paradox, fasting is part and parcel of healthy eating habits. Not only does it stimulate autophagy and body cleansing by destroying old cells and other junk, it also stimulates growth hormone, which tells your body to start producing new cells. What is actually happening during a fast, is that your body is being "revamped" inside-out.

Intermittent fasting, strongly recommended by Dr. Gundry, is very beneficial: it *improves your heart health, increases your brain function, prevents many chronic diseases, and increases your lifespan.*

This way of fasting focuses on alternating between periods of eating normally, and periods of abstaining from food. There are many variations of intermittent fasting diets, and you should choose the one that best fits your lifestyle.

3 common ways of intermittent fasting:

Alternate day fasting

Fasting every other day and eating to satisfaction on the other days.

One day per week fasting

The one day per week fast allows your body to rest and cleanse itself from the rich and toxin-laden diet.

Eating windows

You give yourself a couple of hours "window" (anything from 2 to 6 hours) during the day when you can eat and abstain from food the rest of the time (you only take water). For example, you break your fast by having some fresh fruit or vegetable, and an hour later have a meal, after which you don't take any food for the next 20 hours.

Fasting for five days a month

Many believe that this is the optimal number of days to fast.

Studies reveal that humans are the only primates who can store fat to use later, and that is believed to be the reason the humans managed to successfully inhabit even the most inhospitable parts of the world. We can eat a lot when food is available, and store surplus as fat, and then use that fat during the lean times of famine, drought or winter.

While we lived in synch with the seasons, we all had this metabolic flexibility and easily accumulated fat, but just as easily burned it for fuel, when food was unavailable. Unfortunately, like so many other instincts and functions, we have lost this survival technique, mainly because food is now available the year round. For long-term good health, it's necessary to regain your ability to burn fat for fuel. In other words, you must develop metabolic flexibility. This allows your cells to switch between using carbohydrates and fat as a fuel source. Once you've regained this ability to burn fat for fuel, you can engage in carb-loading once or twice a week.

This means that while you should eat according to Plant Paradox dietary regime most of the time, once or twice a week treat yourself to eating as many carbohydrates as you want to. However, remember that these must be healthy, and if possible lectin-free carbohydrates.

Those who manage to regain their metabolic flexibility will perform better under duress. Even if exposed to extreme conditions and pressure, they will be much less likely to get tired easily, because they will simply tap into their source of fat for an additional energy boost.

Another activity Dr. Gundry strongly recommends for optimal health is following seasonal clocks. This means eating more at times of plenty (i.e. in summer), while practicing intermittent fasting during winter months, to mimic the ancient rhythm of food availability. Dr. Gundry fasts intermittently for six months a year, breaking his fast on 1 June.

Eat according to PP Food Pyramid

The first food pyramid was published in Sweden in 1974. The 1992 US issued a food pyramid called "Food Guide Pyramid" which was updated in 2005, only to be replaced in 2011 by MyPlate chart. However, even that one is already considered outdated.

What all food pyramids have in common is food groups, specifying what percentage of what food should be used in a diet.

There are different types of food pyramids, e.g.: Vegetarian food pyramid, Mediterranean food pyramid, UK: The Eatwell plate, China: Food guide pagoda, France: Ascending steps to health, etc.

The Plant Paradox food pyramid differs considerably from all of these. Its approach to what is healthy is based on the idea that no lectin-rich foods should be allowed on your plate and that most of your diet should consist of vegetables and good fats.

The base of the pyramid is its biggest section and consists of leafy and cruciferous vegetables and good fats.

These are considered the most important dietary ingredients which we should eat the most of.

Don't eat anything

Going without food from time to time gives your body a break and is in line with the idea of intermittent fasting.

Nuts, flour alternatives, lectin-free grains and resistant starches

This is the next biggest section and is, probably, the most difficult one to adjust to.

Wild-caught seafood, pastured poultry and Omega-3 eggs and in-season fruit

Because of its high glucose content, fruit should be treated as a healthy kind of sweet and eaten only a couple of times a week.

Southern European cow's, goat's, sheep's and buffalo milk and red wine, champagne and dark spirits

Only certain kinds of dairy products are safe to eat. Red wine was added because it's known to have many health benefits.

Grass-fed, pasture-raised meat

Unlike the government-recommended food pyramid where meat represents the foundation of the pyramid, i.e. its largest section, with the Plant Paradox diet you don't have to give up meat but can consume only the best quality and only in very small quantities.

Eat (and live) in tune with the seasons

Fruit, because of its high sugar content, is allowed only occasionally, not more than a couple of times a week. However, once you rekindle your metabolism and activate your metabolic flexibility, you can eat fruit freely on your carb-load days.

One thing Dr. Gundry insists on is to eat only fruit that is in season, for that is the only time when its lectin levels are very low. In other words, fruit is no longer trying to protect itself from being eaten by a predator.

On the contrary, it wants to be eaten so that its seed has a chance to sprout in another location.

This is how fruit was eaten in pre-agriculture times – once a year when it was in season. Today, fruit from all over the world is available all the time. Unfortunately, that means that most of it was picked while it was still green, i.e. full of lectins, and forced to ripen with the use of chemicals. Such fruit (and most of the fruit we eat is like that) is full of lectins and potentially harmful, especially to those with a sensitive digestive system.

So, once you start burning your fat for fuel, you are free to gorge on local, seasonal fruit during the summer months, preparing yourself for the lean months of winter, when intermittent fasting will keep you tuned-in with Nature.

Yes foods, No foods, and Alternatives

The food choices of the Plant Paradox diet is what makes it so special. Foods approved by this regime should all be lectin-free.

The most lectin-rich foods are potatoes, eggplants, tomatoes, peppers, kidney beans, lima beans, lentils, wheat, corn, soybean, peanuts, cashews, sunflower seed, goji berries, squash.

Does this mean you should never eat them? In theory, you shouldn't, but in real life, this may be difficult to stick to for long. Partly because these are staple foods from Peking to New York, and partly because many of these foods are important ingredients in cooking.

But, don't worry. The Plant Paradox diet is not that restrictive. Only those with autoimmune disorders and serious gut problems must stick to Plant Paradox regime all the time. Others can use even lectin-rich foods, but prepare them in a way that will reduce, or destroy the lectin.

However, even if you are lectin-intolerant and you occasionally use lectin-rich foods, it won't kill you. You may, or may not, experience digestive problems, and if you do, all you need to do for the problem to go away is remove such food from your diet.

On the other hand, many people tolerate lectin quite well, and if you are one of them, try to process the food you eat in a way that will remove most of the lectins, but how far you'll go with this, is up to you.

Yes Foods

1.   The first layer consists of foods that should be the most prominent in your diet, e.g. broccoli, cauliflower, Brussel sprouts, bok choy, cabbage, asparagus, radish, avocado, lettuce, kohlrabi, spinach, parsley, fennel, seaweed. For seasoning and cooking, you can use extra virgin olive oil, avocado oil, walnut oil, sesame oil and coconut oil.

2.   The second layer is left empty which means you should periodically abstain from food. Try to follow an intermittent fasting method that least disrupts your lifestyle.

3.   The third layer consists of nuts and flour alternatives which can be consumed daily, but within limit, e.g.: macadamia, walnut, pistachios, pecans, coconut, hazelnut, chestnut.

As flour alternatives, you can use coconut flour or almond flour. The only two approved grains are millet and sorghum, both of which are lectin-free and very nutritious. Resistant starches are also included here because they feed friendly bacteria in the gut. They can be found in green bananas and plantains.

4.   The fourth layer consists of wild-caught fish, very rich in important nutrients, and pastured poultry, a healthy source of protein. A modest portion of fruit every day is OK provided it's in season.

Fruits that are OK to eat the year round, provided they are not fully ripened, are mangos, papayas, avocado, and banana. If they are unripe, their sugar content is low.

5.   The fifth layer is milk. Casein-A1 type milk is the milk we consume, but this is, unfortunately, a very unhealthy food choice, mainly due to overuse of growth-hormones. It's known to be able to prompt an immune attack and cause all kinds of other problems. If possible, try to switch to the Southern European type of dairy products, but use them in moderation.

The red wine was included in this section because it contains some very healthy nutrients, but even though it's healthy, it should be consumed only a couple of times a week.

6.   The sixth layer is the smallest section of this pyramid and it includes grass-fed, pasture-raised meats, e.g.: bison, wild game, venison, boar, elk, port, lamb, beef.

No Foods

Unfortunately, foods to be avoided is what we eat most of. They are not only unhealthy, they are often a direct cause of obesity, arthritis or fatigue, and it's best to avoid them.

- Refined starches: potatoes, rice, wheat (including all wheat products, e.g. flour, cereal, pastries)
- Sugar and sweeteners: sugar, agave, honey, maple syrup, aspartame
- Certain fruits and vegetables: legumes, squash, tomatoes, melon, courgettes, peppers, goji berries, lentils
- Soy products: soy, tofu, edamame, soy sauce
- Dairy: Non-Southern European cow milk products, yogurt, ice cream, ricotta, cottage cheese, kefir

- Seeds: Pumpkin, chia and sunflower seeds, peanuts and cashew nuts
- Oils: soy, grapeseed, corn, peanut, cottonseed, sunflower, canola oil
- Grains: oats, whole grains, quinoa, rye, barley, buckwheat, corn, spelt

Alternatives

Dr. Gundry gives an extensive list of permitted and forbidden foods in his book and you should, whenever possible, try to stick to those he recommends in his Food Pyramid. However, not everyone may have access to tapioca flour, plantain, Southern European goat's milk yogurt, or sorghum.

The way to approach the Plant Paradox diet is to grasp the basics and not get put off if you can't get or afford certain recommended foods.

5 things to consider when thinking about going on this diet:

1. What attracts you to this diet? Do you know (or suspect) you are lectin-intolerant and would like to try lectin-free diet? Are you concerned with the general state of your health and would like to improve it by adopting healthy eating habits, even though you have no problem digesting lectin? Have you been struggling with an auto-immune disease for years and see this as an opportunity to help yourself?
2. Study the recommended lists of Yes and No foods and figure out how much of this food is available locally and if you can afford it.
3. In case you don't have access to some of the foods strongly recommended by Plant Paradox pyramid, try to find out what the alternatives are. The most challenging bit is finding the alternative for flour. There are ways of making very nice bread with almond and coconut flour, or tapioca or plantain, although this may take time getting used to.

4. Many other foods which are not on the NO list contain lectins, however, even if you decide to follow this diet, don't become obsessed with lectins. Unless you are ill, you don't have to follow it to the letter. In fact, many people tolerate lectin quite well, so if you are one of them, try to avoid lectin in your diet when you can, and learn about food preparation methods which reduce or even destroy lectins in food.

5. There are many local foods which are not on the Plant Paradox list, but which you can use as an alternative. Be creative and listen to your body. Foods that always give you gas and indigestion are obviously not good for you, so either excludes them from your diet or learn alternative ways of preparing them. Feel free to continue using foods that may contain lectin, but which you digest without a problem. The main items to try and stay away from are grains and legumes.

PART 3

PUTTING IT ALL TOGETHER

Chapter 5

Plant Paradox Diet

Create your Plant Paradox diet plan

When creating your own diet plan, ignore the trendy eating plans and choose a diet that works for YOU. A successful diet should address your nutritional requirements, your lifestyle, and your preferences.

8 steps for creating a personalized Plant Paradox diet plan:

Understand what Plant Paradox is all about

If you decided to adopt the Plant Paradox principles, or at least include some of them into your eating plan, make sure you understand what this diet is about and why so many foods need to be excluded from it.

Understand your own nutritional requirements

Before going on a diet, and particularly before going on a diet which is drastically different from the way you've been eating until now, consider your age, your profession, your geographical environment, your health, and anything else that might affect your personal nutritional needs.

The dietary requirements of a 25-year old are very different from those of a middle-aged person. Your gender, constitution, profession as well as the environment you live in (Australian and Norwegian environments require a different calorie intake), all play a part when deciding what diet to choose and how to approach creating your personalized diet plan.

Understand your lifestyle requirements

Your lifestyle is often what decides if you'll manage to stick to a diet or not. Some popular diets seem to have been created only for those who stay at home, or who work from home, or who can afford to spend their entire day drinking freshly-squeezed vegetable juices, eating special meals, exercising and going for a detox massage.

Before going on a diet, study its main arguments and try to figure out if you can fit those into your lifestyle. If you work long hours and get home late, chances are you are probably so exhausted by the time you get home, the last thing you need is to cook. In that case, you can either prepare most of the meals on weekend, and then simply warm them up when you are ready to eat. Or, you can structure your diet in such a way that it revolves around vegetable salads and other greens which don't require long preparation time.

On the other hand, if you stay at home, or work from home, you can always find time to prepare fresh, healthy, home-cooked meals.

If you often dine out, you'll have to learn what food to order so that your nights out don't disrupt your healthy eating habits. If you travel a lot, it probably means you eat between meetings or flights. In that case, ensure you always have some healthy snacks in your bag, desk, or a car.

Set goals

Many people will only persevere with a certain task if they have a final goal, i.e. if they know what they have set out to achieve. When it comes to a diet, that goal is usually weight loss, which is measurable. But, if your goal is achieving a healthy lifestyle, that may only become obvious after a while, when others start complementing not only on your weight, but complexion, quality of hair, or positive mood.

Remember that even the most challenging task is easier to handle if you know why you are doing it.

Make a diet plan

Why have you chosen this diet? Once you know that, navigating your way through it will be easier. Besides, a diet is not just eating habit, it usually means a lifestyle change too. Plant Paradox is a unique and very different approach to food, and because it excludes most of the foods we consider our staple diet (e.g. wheat, rice, beans) or foods we enjoy very much (e.g. sweets, cakes, biscuits, ice-cream, dairy, etc.), adopting it requires some forward planning.

The best way to plan a diet is to make sure you believe in its philosophy. If you do, it will be so much easier to accept even the difficult parts. Can you "see" yourself eating and living the way the diet requires? Can you "see" yourself benefiting from this eating plan? Do you think it all makes sense? If you answered YES to all these questions, then you're on the right track.

Create a menu

It will save you a lot of time, and help you stick to your diet if you are more or less clear about what you need to have for each meal. This also helps with shopping, for you won't buy foods you no longer need, or which might be too tempting to keep at home.

The best way to start creating a menu is to figure out what you would be needing for the most important meal of the day. Depending on your lifestyle, it could be breakfast, lunch or dinner. Or, if you enjoy snacking throughout the day, first figure out what are the approved snacks and stock up on those.

Make a list of recipes you will use for each meal. You can download them from the Internet, copy them from Dr. Gundry's book or create your own. If you decide to stick to the Plant Paradox diet, some of the foods you will now have to start using instead of flour could be new to you. Find out about all flour alternatives and if they are available locally. If they are not, find out what is.

Once you know what you'll be eating, start figuring out the way the new diet requires food to be prepared – is it mainly raw foods, or cooked, or both.

Create a weekly or monthly shopping list

This makes shopping easy and quick. Foods that can be stored (e.g. oil, millet, honey) you can buy monthly, while fruit and vegetable can be bought on the weekly basis. Find out about local organic markets and health shops.

Learn healthy cooking methods

If you don't like or don't have time to cook, now is the time to learn some basic cooking skills. Fortunately, healthy eating habits usually require food to be processed as little as possible, so you won't have to spend a lot of time in the kitchen.

If you find it difficult to accept all Plant Paradox approved foods, it's OK to cheat a little, until you get used to new tastes and foods.

3 things to bear in mind when creating a Plant Paradox diet plan:

Certain foods should be avoided

The main philosophy of the Plant Paradox diet is to abstain from lectin-rich food. This means no grains, no legumes. This may take time getting used to, but if you find this too challenging, adopt this diet gradually, slowly giving up lectin-rich foods, one at a time, while at the same time slowly introducing new lectin-free foods into your diet.

There are also foods that should be avoided because of the way they are produced. However, certain foods are not bad *per se*. There is a link between Western farm-raised meat, eggs, and grains and chronic diseases. So, buy pasture-raised or wild-caught meat and organic eggs. That way, you won't have to give up meat and eggs, if you think you need them in your diet.

If you can't give up lectin-rich foods, learn how to reduce or destroy their lectin

a) When it comes to legumes, the best way to reduce the lectin is to soak them overnight prior to cooking and cook them thoroughly.

b) The most efficient way of destroying the lectins of beans, tomatoes or potatoes is by pressure cooking. Unfortunately, lectins in wheat, oats, rye, barley, or spelt can't be destroyed this way, so it's best to avoid those entirely. Pressure cooking works only with certain vegetables and legumes.

c) If using some of the lectin-rich vegetables, it's best to peel and deseed them (cucumbers, eggplant, and squash). The hull, peel or rind is the most lectin-filled part of any plant.

d) Fermentation significantly reduces lectins in fruit and vegetable, because it allows the good bacteria to break down and convert lectins and other damaging substances.

e) If you can't give up grain, use refined flour rather than whole grain.

The seed of tomato and cucumber, the skin of eggplant and cucumber, the hull of brown rice or whole wheat, are not toxic enough to kill you, but just enough to cause some serious digestive disorders. Avoid them.

Plant Paradox diet may seem very restrictive at first, but once you study it carefully you'll realize that with a little bit of forward planning, it's a relatively easy way to protect your immune system and digestive organs.

Fasting Paradox

Fasting is often used to restore health when everything else has failed. From this, we can assume that this is something people will engage in as the last resort. However, it hasn't always been like that.
People have regularly used fasting for spiritual or physical cleansing for thousands of years. Unfortunately, we now regard this practice as something one does in desperation. This is one of the examples how modern lifestyle and eating habits have made us turn our back on an ancient, time-tested healing method. On the other hand, animals have not lost this knowledge and abstain from food whenever they are not feeling well. We, usually, do the opposite.

As Dr. Gundry points out in his Plant Paradox pyramid, abstaining from food is essential for optimal health. Something we often forget is that for tens of thousands of years, humans survived successfully on irregular, and uncertain food supply. When food was plentiful they feasted, when it was scarce they fasted. Sometimes they starved. However, this is not as horrible as it sounds. Humans and animals both can survive on very little or no food for even couple of months because the body stores nutrients in the fat, blood, bone marrow and other tissues. Nature equipped us with a phenomenal surviving mechanism, which we, unfortunately, allowed to decline and disappear.

Holistic medicine has always regarded fasting as very beneficial because it gives your body a chance to rest, and in the process, get rid of toxins that have accumulated for years.

4 reasons we have become so unhealthy:

- We eat much more than we need
- We eat all the time
- We eat unhealthy foods
- We lead sedentary lifestyles

Reasons for these unhealthy living habits are many, but they all revolve around the Western diet:

- Today, food is, generally speaking, plentiful, particularly in the developed world. And thanks to modern agriculture practices, it's cheap.
- Agriculture is a million-dollar business, and aggressive marketing campaigns encourage people to eat a lot, to eat all the time and to eat processed foods.
- Processed foods are usually very tasty because they are full of salt, sugar and flavor additives.
- Processed foods are addictive.
- The so-called Western diet is very rich in calories which you can only burn if you are involved in strenuous exercise (which most of us are not), or if you starve (which most of us don't). The sedentary lifestyle turns most of the food we consume into fat and starts storing it, starting with the waistline.

There is a parallel between sleep and fasting. If you deprive yourself of sleep for a long time, your system will eventually break down. Something similar happens with your digestive system – unless you give it a rest from time to time, it becomes clogged with yeasts, acid wastes, undigested foods and various toxins.

The best thing about fasting is that it's a relatively easy way to counter effect the consequences of the modern diet.

8 ways fasting improves your health:

- It cleanses the body of accumulated toxins
- It gives you more energy because the energy needed for digestion is redirected to other tasks, such as repair and heal the body
- Blood pressure normalizes
- Immune system is boosted
- Blood sugar level normalizes
- Inflammatory processes subside
- Blood flow increase, as arteries widen
- Inflammation of skin, bladder, and bowl subside

However, people fast not just for health reasons, but for religious (e.g. Muslims during the festival of Ramadan), and spiritual ones as well (many yogis fast twice a month on "Ekadasi" days, the 11th and 22nd lunar days of the month which are considered especially auspicious for the practice of fasting).

One thing I noticed during my first fast, was how much free time I suddenly had. Only then did I realize how much time we spend on food-related activities: shopping for food, preparing the food for cooking, cooking it, laying the table, eating, washing up, etc.

Another thing I noticed was the surplus of energy. To say that fasting made me feel more energized would be putting it mildly. I felt lighter, as well as brighter. It seems that just 5 days of juice fast invigorated my body so much, that I felt I could move mountains. What was also surprising was that I not only didn't need coffee or tea during the day, I couldn't bring myself to drink anything except juice and water.

Three most common ways to fast:

Juice fast

Depending on whether you are fasting as part of an anti-cancer treatment, or for a general detox, you will use different vegetables and fruits for your juices.

Water fast

This is the so-called total fast, i.e. when you abstain from all food, solid or liquid. Water is not a food. It's important to drink plenty of water during a fast as it helps to cleanse the body and flush the toxins out of the system. Water fasting can last up to 3, 5, 10, 20, and even 40 days.

Intermittent Fasting

Intermittent fasting can be done in many ways. For example, you may decide to abstain from food for 12, or 36 hours a day. Dr. Gundry recommends "seasonal" intermittent fasting, to bring ourselves in line with natural cycles.

Since food was probably scarce during the winter months, we assume hunter-gatherers often went without food for days, for in winter there were no roots, tubers, fruits or nuts to carry them thorough meatless days. Therefore, Dr. Gundry recommends (and personally practices) a 36-hour fast for six months a year, breaking the fast on 1 June, when, in synch with the season of plenty, he resumes more regular eating.

Things to know about fasting

First 24-hours of fasting, the body burns glucose present in the bloodstream, and hunger occurs.

24 – 48 hours, the burns glycogen from muscles and tissues.

3 days and beyond into fasting, the body starts to burn fat. Hunger seems to go away, most of the time at least as some may still experience hunger. During the 3rd day and beyond, the body starts it detoxification process and eventually healing process.

When and how long to fast

- If you are new to fasting, it's best to begin with a short fast. You can safely do one-day fast once a week or choose one of the intermittent fasting methods.
- Fasting on a regular basis will prolong your physical and mental fitness.
- Weekend fasts are recommended several times per year, especially at the times when the seasons are changing.
- Hunger usually disappears after the third day of a long fast.

Possible side effects

- The tongue may feel furry while fasting. You can use a tongue cleanser to remove the toxins that exit the body via the tongue, or you may choose to brush your teeth and rinse your mouth frequently.
- Some people, especially those new to fasting, experience a headache or nausea. Should that happen, have some hot peppermint tea. Don't take ordinary tea or coffee.
- After three days, peristaltic action will slow down and stop in the small intestine, which may lead to constipation. That's why many recommend the daily use of an enema.
- You may feel cold, so try to keep yourself warm throughout the fast. For this reason, it's easier to fast during summer.
- You may become over-sensitive, as the fast also helps cleanse the emotional toxins (e.g. unresolved issues or feeling you keep bottled up).

When and how to break the fast

During the time we spend sleeping, our body is resting from food. Breakfast (break – fast), as the name implies, is a meal that breaks a nightly fast. As fast is a detoxification process, you shouldn't be surprised if upon waking up you experience heavy breath, coated tongue, blurry mind – these are all signs your body has undergone a brief detoxification process.

Breaking a fast, especially a long one, needs to be done properly. If you've been fasting several weeks on water or juice, don't take heavy food as soon as you break the fast. Continue to drink water or juice while introducing a vegetable salad for lunch and maybe a fruit in the afternoon. After a couple of days, add a steamed vegetable to your diet. Gradually, return to a balanced diet, trying to exclude unhealthy foods. After a long rigorous fast, you need to give your body at least ten days to adjust to solid foods.

As Swami Sivananda pointed out in one of his lectures, "Both fasting and feasting are blessings to human beings. The feast gives you an immediate blessing, which vanishes in a few hours, inducing a craving for more, whereas a fast gives you a different kind of happiness, more lasting than a feast".

CAUTION

If you are on medications that can't be stopped, you should not take fasting.

Although fasting is an excellent remedy, it cannot cure deficiency diseases that result from insufficient nourishment or congenital defects. Do not fast if you are pregnant, if you suffer from anemia or diabetes, or if you had had an eating disorder.

74

Chapter 6

Plant Paradox Eating Plan

Plant Paradox diet shopping list

Food is part of our culture, much more than we realize. Just like in Asia they can't imagine a meal without rice, in Northern Europe diets revolve around potatoes and dairy, in the Middle East around bread and vegetable, and in Africa around corn, sorghum or millet.

Well, if you decide to eat according to the Plant Paradox principles, all that is about to change. The Plant Paradox highlights the potential, and often real, havoc that lectin-rich foods can wreak on your digestive and immune system.

Adopting this diet requires that you give up almost everything you ate most of until now, e.g. rice, wheat, potatoes, beans, dairy, etc. When I first found out about this die, I wondered what these could be replaced with, but with a bit of research, I realized that things are not as bleak as they seem.

Although almost all foods contain lectin to a certain degree, which means that even if you are lectin-intolerant you would still not be able to eat only lectin-free foods, certain food preparation methods can help you reduce or even destroy the lectin.

If you've been eating a typical Western diet so far, I hope you realize that your diet is going to be drastically different from what it used to be. However, if you ate a healthy diet, then you won't find the new eating habits that difficult to adjust to. From now on, your staple diet should be millet, coconut, and almond. When it comes to vegetables, again, the most popular ones, such as tomatoes, peppers, courgettes, should be avoided.

There are a lot of lectin-free recipes available on the Internet and in Dr. Gundry's book, so the ones I included in this book, are just a few to give you an idea of what sort of meals you should be eating, and to get you started on your new diet. If you enjoy cooking and experimenting with new recipes, you'll enjoy this. If you don't, you can focus on eating fresh vegetable salads and soups, as these are easy to prepare.

Those who tolerate lectin well, can continue to use the lectin-rich foods, but use them less than they used to, and always peel, deseed or soak them, prior to use.

However, let's be realistic. Unless you're allergic to lectin or have a serious lectin-related disease, chances are you will not stick to this diet all the time. So, let's look at the real-life situations. You need to be resourceful and creative, rather than become obsessed with following the Plant Paradox instructions to the letter.

How to use "forbidden" foods:

- Substitute dairy with goat-milk or sheep-milk products
- Soak beans overnight, changing the water several times, and cook them thoroughly
- Avoid bell peppers as they seem to be particularly rich in lectin
- Ferment vegetables that can be fermented
- Peel and deseed cucumber, tomato, courgette, eggplant

- Potatoes should always be peeled and cooked well. Never eat potatoes whose skin has gone green, for even heat can't destroy these toxins.

-

Foods that in my opinion are most difficult to give up, or replace, are bread and rice. Many of the recipes listed in Dr. Gundry's book that could replace grains are plantain, tapioca, green bananas, and sorghum. Unfortunately, these may not be available to everyone, so I suggest you base your new diet on foods which are available everywhere throughout the year: millet, coconut, and almond.

Millet

Millet is an ancient crop that has been grown in Asia and Africa for over 10,000 years. It's an alkaline food and is easy to digest. Hulled millet is an excellent source of very important minerals, such as copper, phosphorus, manganese, and magnesium. It's also rich in prebiotic dietary fiber. Millet is easy to prepare and quick to cook and is a perfect substitution for grains, rice, and pasta.

Millet can be cooked in two ways:

If cooked in plenty of water it becomes creamy like mashed potatoes, and can be used for stuffings, burgers, and toppings on vegetables.

If roasted first, and cooked with a little less water, the result is a fluffy grain like couscous and cooked this way it can replace rice in most recipes.

Coconut

Because of its amazing nutritional and healing properties, coconut and all its products - coconut flesh, coconut water, coconut oil, and coconut cream - is considered one of the most amazing plants of all time.

Because of its strong antioxidant properties and health benefits, the coconuts can be used to:

- Lower cholesterol
- Improve digestion
- Ward off wrinkles
- Kill bacteria and viruses
- Lose weight
- Increase metabolism

When baking with coconut flour, don't forget that you should use almost twice as many eggs as you would if you were cooking with wheat flour. This is because coconut flour is extremely absorbent and requires a high ratio of liquid ingredients to flour.

Almond

Almonds are packed with vitamins, minerals, protein, and fiber, and are known to be one the healthiest of nuts.

Almonds have many health benefits and should be part of everyone's diet:

- They can help prevent heart attack
- They improve brain function
- They maintain skin health
- They can prevent diabetes and help control blood sugar levels
- They improve digestion

They are best raw, whole or ground, provided they are skinned, for that's where lectins hide. Use them as snacks, in salads, in muesli or as flour for bread or cakes.

When it comes to starchy vegetables, the only one with a high percentage of lectins are potatoes. Sweet potatoes and yams also have some lectin, but the good news is that lectin is concentrated in the skin, so peeling potatoes, sweet potatoes, and yams could solve the problem.

Although Dr. Gundry forbids potato and other roots, since most hunter-gatherers ate tubers regularly, they are probably OK to include in a diet, provided the skin is removed. If you catch yourself panicking which food is safe to use and which isn't, since it seems that most of the foods we eat contain a certain amount of lectin, just remember that not all lectin is bad, and even allowed vegetables, e.g. spinach, have them.

The long and short of this diet is to avoid grains, while all other foods can be made lectin-free with suitable preparation methods.

Shopping list

Before making a shopping list for the new diet, study the recommended recipes in this book as well as other lectin-free recipes to get an idea of what sort of foods you'll be using.

Start by asking yourself what you need for a Plant Paradox breakfast. If you are one of those people for whom it's the main meal of the day, you'll need to stock up on pastured-eggs, goat-milk or sheep-milk yogurt and a selection of approved fruit and seed. Otherwise, you'll need lots of millet, almond, coconut and healthy oils. However, the most important ingredient of your diet should be vegetables, particularly the cruciferous ones.

Basically, you need to stock up on:

- Vegetables (fresh or frozen). This should be the main component of your diet and it should represent about 50% of your meal. Cruciferous vegetables are the best, e.g. cabbage, cauliflower, Brussels sprouts, broccoli, etc.
- Good fats (oils): olive, avocado, walnut, sesame and coconut oils should be your only source of fats.
- Plant Paradox approved nuts: macadamia, walnuts, almonds, pecans, pistachios, and hazelnut to snack on if you feel hungry between meals or to add to salads or cereal.

- As a starch substitute, you can use coconut, almond, and millet, and all your breads and cakes should be made from these.
- Fish, if you eat it. Choose wild-caught if you can.
- Fruit, only seasonal and only couple of times a week.
- Milk and dairy products should be used in small quantities, and even so only as yogurt which, being fermented is very healthy and contains good probiotics. However, either buy Casein A2-type of dairy or go for goat and sheep milk products.
- Finally, you can eat a little bit of meat, but only pasture-raised or wild-caught because meat raised by conventional methods is far too toxic to be healthy.
- Sugar should be avoided, or at least reduced, and you can use honey instead.

Buy organic, whenever you can.

Plant Paradox Menu

These are just a few ideas of what to eat on the Plant Paradox diet. Get creative and develop your own recipes. If you're new to cooking or if you don't enjoy it or don't have time for it, focus on salads and steamed vegetable. The healthiest meals are those prepared simply, with as little processing as possible.

I included only vegetarian recipes, but if you eat meat, you are free to add pasture-raised or wild-caught meats and fish to your diet.

Breakfast

- Fruit salad with seed mix
- Millet muesli
- Nut-and-seed muesli
- Smoothies
- Toast and nut butter

- Muffins with fruit juice
- Pancakes with berries
- Dried fruit coconut cereal
- Almond muffins with seasonal fruit
- Mushroom and spinach frittata
- Pumpkin bread with goat-milk yogurt

Snacks

- Fruit with a handful of almonds
- Crudities with dip
- Avocado with lemon juice
- Fruit with a handful of nuts
- Fruit and seed mix
- Olives
- Handful of mixed nuts (almonds, walnuts, pine nuts, macadamia)
- Pomegranate or grapefruit
- Apple with handful of walnuts
- Juice and nuts

Lunch

- Vegetable salad with seed mix (or nuts)
- Trout with roasted vegetables
- Pumpkin bread and vegetable spread
- Soup with bread
- Goat-milk cheese sandwich with lots of greens
- Roasted vegetables drizzled with honey (this goes well with sweetish-tasting vegetables such as carrots and sweet potatoes)

Starters

- Olive spread
- Celeriac root pate
- Mushroom pate
- Miso nut spread
- Coconut chutney
- Stuffed button mushrooms
- Summer millet salad

Dinner

- Chestnut roast and romaine salad
- Savory millet cakes and artichoke salad
- Mushroom and pine nut stuffed courgettes with mixed salad
- Salad of quinoa and roasted vegetables
- Carrots Algerian style with grilled mushrooms
- Millet stirfry with spinach-and-avocado salad
- Millet "pillau"
- Steamed vegetables with coconut chutney
- Millet "couscous" with vegetables
- Cauliflower curry with millet

Desert

- Wine-stewed fresh figs
- Raisin coconut balls
- Sesame balls
- Fruit salad
- Moroccan fruit cups
- Roasted apples drizzled with honey

Plant Paradox Diet Recipes

Breakfast ideas

Millet muesli

- 2 tbsp ground millet
- 1 tbsp sunflower seed
- 1 tbsp flax seed, ground
- 1 apple, grated or 1 cup berries in season
- 1 tbsp raisin
- lemon juice
- 1 tbsp almond butter, or 1 tbsp olive oil, or 1 tbsp flax seed oil
- 1 banana
- 1 tbsp walnuts, ground
- Goat-milk yogurt, or grated apple

Mix all the ingredients, and sprinkle with ground walnuts. You can mix in some goat-milk yogurt or a grated apple.

Dried fruit coconut cereal

- 2 cups pecans chopped
- $1/3$ cup coconut oil
- 6 medium dates, pitted
- 1 cup almonds, roughly chopped
- 1 tablespoon vanilla
- 2 teaspoons cinnamon
- $1/2$ teaspoon sea salt
- $1/2$ cup coconut flakes

- $^1/_2$ cup dried apricots

Preheat oven.

Put half the pecans, coconut oil, and dates in a food processor, or chop finely.

Add the remaining pecans and almonds.

Transfer to a bowl and add the vanilla, cinnamon, and salt. Stir and spread on a baking sheet. Bake for about 20 minutes, until browned. Remove, let cool, and stir in the coconut flakes and apricots.

Store in an airtight container.

Nut-and-seed muesli

- 1 cup almonds whole or slivered
- 1 cup pecans roughly chopped
- 2 cup walnuts roughly chopped
- 2 tablespoons chia seeds
- 2 tablespoons flax seeds, ground
- 2 tablespoons coconut oil melted
- 1 tablespoon honey
- $^1/_2$ teaspoon cinnamon
- 1 cup raisins
- 1 cup blueberries

Preheat oven.

In a large mixing bowl, combine almonds, pecans, walnuts, sunflower seeds, chia, flax, coconut oil, honey, and cinnamon. Stir with a wooden spoon to coat.

Spread mixture evenly on a baking tray. Bake, stirring occasionally, for about 20 minutes.

Remove from oven and cool 5 minutes. Add raisins and blueberries and stir to combine.

Serve with almond or coconut milk. To store, cool muesli completely and keep in an airtight container at room temperature.

Apple Cinnamon Muffins

- 2 small apples, diced
- 1 tablespoon lemon juice
- 5 large eggs
- $1/2$ cup coconut flour
- 2 tablespoons cinnamon
- $1/8$ teaspoon nutmeg, ground
- 1 teaspoon baking soda
- 4 tablespoon coconut oil melted
- $1/4$ teaspoon salt

Preheat oven. Grease a muffin tin.

Put the apples in a saucepan with the lemon juice and cover. Add enough water to cover half. Bring to a boil, reduce heat and simmer for 10 minutes, until apples are broken down. Transfer to a blender and puree until smooth. Leave to cool for 5 minutes. While apples are still warm, add the remaining ingredients to the blender and puree on low until you have a thick batter.

Pour the batter into your prepared muffin tin, filling each tin about 3/4 full. Bake for about 15 minutes, until tops are firm. Cool before removing from pan.

Carrot banana muffin

- 2 cups almond flour
- 2 teaspoons baking soda
- $1/2$ teaspoon sea salt
- 1 tablespoon cinnamon
- 1 cup dates, pitted
- 3 medium bananas
- 3 large eggs
- 1 teaspoon apple cider vinegar
- $1/4$ cup coconut oil melted
- $1\,1/2$ large carrots shredded
- $3/4$ cup walnuts, finely chopped

Preheat oven.

In a large bowl, combine flour, baking soda, salt, and cinnamon.

In a food processor, combine dates, bananas, eggs, vinegar, and oil.

Add mixture from food processor to dry mixture in the large bowl and combine thoroughly.

Fold in carrots and nuts.

Spoon mixture into paper lined muffin tins.

Bake at medium temperature for 25 minutes.

Almond flour pancakes

- 1 cup almond flour
- $1/2$ cup applesauce, unsweetened
- 1 tablespoon coconut flour

- 2 large eggs
- $1/4$ cup water
- $1/4$ teaspoon nutmeg, fresh
- $1/4$ teaspoon salt
- 1 tablespoon coconut oil divided
- $1/2$ cup berries, fresh

Combine almond flour, applesauce, coconut flour, eggs, water, nutmeg and sea salt in a bowl, and mix together completely with a fork. The batter will appear a little thicker than a normal mix.

Heat a non-stick frying pan over medium-low heat with coconut oil.

Drop 1/4 cup of batter onto the pan once it is fully heated. Spread out batter slightly if desired.

Flip like a normal pancake when the bubbles start showing up on the top and cook for another minute or two.

Add more oil to the pan and repeat with remaining batter.

Top with fresh berries.

Banana-berry-flax seed smoothie

- 1 banana
- 1 cup berries, seasonal
- 2 tablespoons ground flax seed
- 1 teaspoon coconut oil
- $1/4$ cup coconut milk, or water

Green smoothie

- 2 apples, quartered

- 2 handfuls of baby spinach, shredded
- 1 handful of parsley (or 2 celery stalks with leaves)
- 1 avocado
- 2 spoons of pine nuts
- 1-2 cups of water

Mushroom and spinach frittata

- 6 large eggs
- $^1/_4$ cup coconut milk
- 250 gr mushrooms, sliced
- 2 cups spinach chopped
- salt and black pepper to taste

Preheat oven.

Whisk the eggs with the coconut milk in a large bowl. Set aside.

Cook the mushroom in olive oil, until all the water evaporates. Drain from oil and set aside.

Add the spinach to the mushroom oil and cook until just wilted. Pour the egg mixture into the skillet and season with salt and pepper.

Bake for 15-20 minutes, until eggs are set.

Decorate with parsley leaves.

Bread Ideas

Pumpkin bread

- 1 cup blanched almond, fine-ground
- $^1/_4$ cup coconut flour
- 1 teaspoon cinnamon

- $^1/_2$ teaspoon baking soda
- $^1/_2$ teaspoon salt
- $^1/_4$ teaspoon cloves, ground
- 1 cup sugar
- $^1/_2$ cup pumpkin puree
- $^1/_3$ cup coconut oil melted
- 3 tablespoons coconut milk
- 1 tsp vanilla extract
- 4 large eggs

Preheat the oven. Line the bottom of a loaf pan with parchment paper.

Combine the flours, cinnamon, baking soda, salt, pumpkin pie spice, cloves, and sugar in the bowl of a large food processor. Mix thoroughly. Then add the pumpkin puree, coconut oil, coconut milk, vanilla bean seeds or extract, and eggs and process for 30 seconds or until combined.

Transfer the mixture to the parchment-lined loaf pan. Bake for 50-60 minutes at medium heat or until a toothpick inserted into the center comes out clean. Let cool in the pan for 15 minutes, before loosening the bread from the pan. Let cool completely before slicing and serving.

Almond coconut bread

- 3 cups almond flour
- 3 tablespoons coconut flour
- 6 tablespoons flax seeds, ground
- $^1/_2$ teaspoon sea salt
- $1^1/_2$ teaspoons baking soda
- 7 large eggs

- $1^1/_2$ tablespoons coconut oil melted

- $1^1/_2$ tablespoons honey, raw

- $1^1/_2$ tablespoons apple cider vinegar

Preheat oven.

In either a food processor or stand mixer, combine the flours, flax, salt and baking soda. Mix until well combined. Add the eggs and beat or pulse until combined. Add the coconut oil, honey and vinegar and mix until well combined.

Lightly coat a standard 9x5 bread pan with coconut oil. Pour the batter in, scraping the sides of the bowl with a spatula.

Bake for 30-40 minutes until the top is browned. Allow to cool.,

Starters Ideas:

Olive spread

- 20 green olives stuffed with pimento
- 2 tablespoons tahini
- 4 tablespoons chopped fresh parsley
- 2 tablespoons extra virgin olive oil

Put all ingredients in a blender and blend to a puree. Alternatively, chop the ingredients very finely. Allow it to set for about 1 hour before serving.

Celeriac pate

- 1 small celeriac (celery root)
- 4 big carrots

- Fresh parsley
- young onion greens
- 1 small red onion
- garlic (optional)
- juice of 1/2 lemon
- salt
- olive oil
- 1 tsp turmeric
- 1/2 cup almond soaked overnight
- 1/2 cup hazelnuts soaked overnight

Put all ingredients in a blender or a food processor but make sure they retain a coarse consistency. Transfer to a bowl, add ground sesame, mix well. You can also add 1/2 ground flax seed. Leave it for 15 minutes for the tastes to develop.

Miso nut spread

- 2 tablespoons hazelnuts or almonds
- 2 tablespoons light miso
- 1 tablespoon water

Roast the nuts in the hot dry frying pan over a high heat until lightly browned. Place them in a blender with the miso and water. Blend together until smooth.

Variation: You can use tahini instead of nuts.

Coconut chutney

- 100 gr desiccated coconut

- 3 tablespoons chopped curry leaves
- 1 cm piece fresh root ginger, peeled and grated
- 1 carrot, grated
- 1 tablespoon coconut oil
- 1 tablespoon black mustard seeds
- 1 tablespoon lemon juice
- 1-2 tablespoons paprika
- 1 tsp salt

Soak the coconut in just enough water to cover it for 15-20 minutes, then squeeze out the liquid. Add the chopped curry leaves, ginger, and carrot. Toss the mixture with your hands until everything is well mixed.

Heat the oil in a frying pan and roast the mustard seeds over a high heat until they "pop". Add the oil and mustard seeds to the coconut mixture and mix well, then stir in the lemon juice, paprika, and salt.

Summer millet salad

For the dressing

- 100 ml olive oil
- 2 tbsp white wine vinegar
- ½ tsp castor sugar
- 2 tsp Dijon mustard
- salt and pepper
- Grated rind of one lemon
- Few snippets of chives (optional)

For the salad:

- 225 gr sun-dried tomatoes
- 1 cup stir-fried and lightly cooked millet
- 225 gr broccoli florets

- 50 gr toasted walnut pieces
- 50 gr pitted black olives
- 200 gr mushrooms, sliced
- 2 hardboiled eggs

Whisk together the dressing ingredients. Fry the thickly sliced mushrooms lightly. Roast the millet, then cook with a little less water than when you normally cook it, to get fluffy grain like couscous.

Steam the broccoli for 2 minutes (you can use it raw if you prefer). Toss all ingredients together. Let stand for 15 minutes before serving.

Goat-milk cheese spread

- 225 gr soft, goat-milk cheese
- 1/2 cup finely chopped olives
- 2 celery ribs, finely chopped
- 2 medium carrots, finely chopped
- 6 radishes, finely chopped
- 4 teaspoons finely chopped onion
- 1 teaspoon dill weed

Vegetable sandwich spread

- ½ cup pickles
- ½ cup olives
- ½ cup onion
- 1 stalk celery
- 3 sun-dried tomatoes
- 225 gr soft, goat-milk cheese
- 2 tsp Worcestershire sauce
- 1 tbsp mayonnaise (optional)
- 1 cup pecans, chopped

- salt, pepper, dried seasoning to taste

Spinach dip

- 250 gr frozen chipped spinach
- 225 gr thick sheep-milk yogurt
- 1 cup mayonnaise
- salt, pepper, dried dill weed to taste
- ¼ cup chopped green onions
- 225 gr water chestnuts, drained, finely chopped
- 50 diced pimientos, drained (optional)

Garlic-chive-yogurt vegetable dip

- 2 medium cloves garlic, minced
- ½ tsp salt
- ½ tsp cayenne pepper
- Black pepper, to taste
- 1 tablespoon chopped chives
- 1 cup sheep-milk yogurt

Black olives and orange salad

- 3 oranges
- 60 gr pitted black olives
- 1 tbsp chopped fresh coriander
- 1 tbsp chopped fresh parsley
- 2 tbsp olive oil
- 1 tsp lemon juice
- 1/2 tsp paprika
- 1/2 tsp ground cumin

Remove the peel and white pith from the oranges and cut into wedges. Place the oranges in the salad bowl, add the black olives, chopped coriander, and parsley. In a small bowl, whisk together the olive oil, lemon juice, paprika, and cumin. Pour the dressing over the salad and toss gently to mix. Chill for 30 minutes before serving.

Millet vegetable salad

- 1 tbsp olive oil
- 5 spring onions, chopped
- 1 garlic clove, crushed
- 1 tsp ground cumin
- 350 ml vegetable stock
- 175 gr millet
- 2 tomatoes skinned, deseeded and finely chopped
- 4 tbsp chopped fresh parsley
- 4 tbsp chopped fresh mint
- 1 green chili, seeded and finely chopped
- 2 tbsp lemon juice
- salt and black pepper
- toasted pine nuts and grated lemon rind to garnish
- crisp lettuce leaves to serve

Heat the oil, add the onions, garlic, and cumin and cook for 1 minute. Add the stock and bring to the boil.

Remove the pan from the heat, stir in the millet, cover the pan and leave it to stand for 10 minutes, or until it has swelled, and all the liquid has been absorbed.

Turn the couscous into a bowl. Stir in the tomatoes, chopped parsley and mint, chili and lemon juice, with salt and pepper to taste. If possible, leave to stand in a cool place for an hour to allow the flavors to develop fully.

To serve, line the bowl with lettuce leaves and spoon the millet salad into the center. Sprinkle the toasted pine nuts and grated lemon rind over, to garnish.

Soups

Leeks soup

- 8 medium leeks, trimmed, leaving white and pale green parts only, and chopped
- 1 medium onion, chopped
- 1 large carrot, chopped
- 2 celery ribs, chopped
- 1 teaspoon salt
- 1/2 teaspoon black pepper
- 1/2 cup unsalted butter
- 1 small boiling potato
- 1/2 cup dry white wine
- 3 cups chicken stock
- 3 cups water
- 1 bay leaf
- 1 ½ cups fresh flat-leaf parsley leaves
- ¼ cup all-purpose flour
- ½ cup sheep-milk yogurt
- 1 tbsp olive oil

Wash sliced leeks and let drain.

Cook leeks, onion, carrot, celery, salt, and black pepper in 4 tablespoons olive oil over moderate heat, stirring occasionally, until softened, about 8 minutes. Peel potato and cut into small cubes, then add to onion mixture along with wine, stock, water, and bay leaf. Bring to a boil, then reduce heat and simmer, partially covered, until vegetables are tender, about 15 minutes.

Stir in parsley and simmer soup, uncovered, 5 minutes. Discard bay leaf and keep soup simmering.

Heat the remaining olive oil then add flour and cook whisking, until golden, about 3 minutes. Remove from heat and add 2 cups simmering stock (from the soup), whisking vigorously, then whisk mixture into remaining soup and return to a simmer, whisking.

Blend soup in 4 batches in a blender until smooth. Season with salt and pepper.

Serve soup topped with thick sheep-milk yogurt.

Cabbage soup

- 4 teaspoons olive oil
- 1/2 teaspoon coriander seeds (or 1/4 teaspoon ground coriander)
- 1/2 teaspoon fennel seeds (or 1/4 teaspoon ground fennel)
- 1/4 teaspoon cumin seeds (or 1/8 teaspoon ground cumin)
- 1 medium onion, chopped
- 1 small cabbage, sliced
- Salt, black pepper to taste
- 300 gr peeled and deseeded tomatoes
- 4 cups chicken stock

Fry dry seed in 2 tbsp olive oil, then add onion, and stir-fry for a couple of minutes, coating it with oil and spice. Add the tomatoes, cabbage and chicken stock. Cook for about 25 minutes.

Carrot soup

- 2 spoonfuls of extra virgin olive oil
- 600 gr carrots, grated
- 500 ml water
- 500 ml orange juice
- salt and pepper
- 2 tablespoons chopped fresh mint

Heat the oil in a large pan and sauté the carrots until they begin to soften. Add the water, half cover and simmer over a low to medium heat for about 20 minutes, until the carrots are soft.

Remove from the heat and allow to cool slightly. Place the carrots and the cooking water in a food processor or a blender, add the orange juice and puree the mixture until smooth. Return the soup to the pan, season to taste with salt and pepper and reheat without boiling. Serve garnished with the chopped mint.

<u>Variation</u>: Omit the orange juice and double the quantity of water. Replace the chopped mint with a pinch of freshly grated nutmeg.

Dinner Ideas

Chestnut roast

- 450 gr fresh chestnuts
- 300 gr mixed nuts (unsalted almond and Brazil nuts are best)
- 200 gr millet
- 650 ml water

- 2 tablespoons extra virgin olive oil
- 2 carrots, grated
- ½ a cabbage, finely sliced
- 2 sticks of celery, chopped
- 250 gr broccoli, broken into florets
- 3 tablespoons tomato puree
- 3 tablespoons tamari
- ¼ tsp pepper
- 1 tablespoon dried mixed herbs
- flaked almonds and parsley sprigs, to garnish

Serve with cranberry sauce.

Preheat the oven. To peel the chestnuts, make a small slit in the pointed end. Place them in a pan, cover with boiling water and leave for 5 minutes. Remove them from the water, one at a time, and peel off the thick outer skin and thin inner skin while warm. Cook the peeled chestnuts in boiling water for about 30 minutes, until soft, and set aside, reserving the water for stock.

Meanwhile, spread out the mixed nuts on a baking sheet and roast in the oven for about 10 minutes, until lightly browned, stirring from time to time. Coarsely chop the nuts and set aside. Cook the millet in the water and set aside.

Heat the oil in a pan and add the carrots, cabbage, and celery. Cover and cook over a medium heat for a few minutes, then add the broccoli and cook for 1-2 minutes. Add the tomato puree, tamari, pepper, mixed herbs, chestnuts, mixed nuts, and cooked millet. Stir in enough reserved stock to bind everything together.

Transfer the mixture to a greased loaf tin and bake it in the oven for about 45 minutes. Garnish with flaked almonds and parsley sprigs and serve with cranberry sauce.

Savory millet cakes

- 400 gr millet
- 900 ml water
- pinch of salt
- 175 gr celery stick or broccoli, chopped
- 3 tsp grated lemon rind
- 3 tablespoons wholemeal flour
- 2 tablespoons extra virgin olive oil
- 200 gr firm tofu crumbled

Place the millet in a large pan with water and salt. Bring to the boil, cover and simmer for 30 minutes. Remove from heat, add the chopped broccoli or celery, cover, and leave to cool. When cold, mash the millet and vegetable. Add the remaining ingredients and stir to make a thick mixture. Add a little extra water if necessary.

Heat oil in a large frying pan. Cook 2 or 3 cakes at a time. To make a cake, place a handful of millet mixture into the pan and press it down with a wet spatula. Cook over a medium heat for 3-4 minutes on each side, until golden brown. Keep warm until they are all cooked.

Serve them with a mixed salad, and steamed vegetables.

Carrots Algerian style

- 1 kg carrots, scraped and cut into 1 cm slices
- 5 tbsp olive oil
- 1 tsp salt
- 1/2 tsp white pepper
- 1/2 tsp ground cinnamon
- 1/2 tsp cumin seeds
- 3 garlic cloves, crushed
- 1/ tsp dried thyme

- 1 bay leaf
- 1 tsp lemon juice

Cook the carrot slices for 15 minutes, or until just tender. Using the slotted spoon, remove them from the pan and transfer them to a bowl. Reserve 150 ml of the cooking liquid.

In a saucepan mix together the oil, salt, pepper, cinnamon, cumin seeds, garlic and thyme over very low heat. Simmer for 10 minutes. Add the reserved cooking liquid and the bay leaf, cover the pan and simmer for further 15 minutes.

Add the carrots to the saucepan. Toss them in the sauce and cook them for 2-3 minutes. Sprinkle them with lemon juice, remove the bay leaf and serve immediately. It can be served cold as well.

Spiced spring carrots

- 4 carrots, cut into matchsticks
- 50 gr flaked almonds
- 5 tablespoons extra virgin olive oil
- 1 tsp ground cumin
- 2 tsp chopped fresh coriander
- 1 tsp clear honey
- salt and pepper

Steam the carrot sticks for 10 minutes, until tender but still crunchy. Meanwhile, set aside a few of the flaked almonds and roast the remainder in a dry heavy pan over a high heat, until golden brown around the edges.

Heat the oil and cook the cumin over a high heat for a few seconds to release the aroma, being careful not to burn them. Take the pan off the heat and add the carrots, browned almonds, and coriander. Mix well then stir in the honey. Add a pinch of salt and pepper. Serve at once, garnished with the reserved almonds.

Millet "stirfry"

- 2 cloves garlic, crushed
- 1 carrot, chopped
- 1 tablespoon olive oil
- 1 onion, chopped
- 5 sun-dried tomatoes, finely chopped
- 1 cup millet
- 2 cups vegetable broth
- salt and ground black pepper to taste
- 1/4 cup chopped fresh cilantro or more to taste

Chop carrot and garlic.

Heat olive oil, cook and stir carrot mixture, onion, and sun-dried tomato until softened, about 10 minutes. Add millet; stir until fragrant and toasted, about 3 minutes.

Pour vegetable broth into millet mixture; season with salt and black pepper. Reduce heat and simmer until all the broth is absorbed and millet is tender, about 20 minutes. Stir in cilantro.

Mushroom-and-pine nut stuffed courgettes

- 4 medium-sized courgettes, peeled, cut in half, lengthwise, and deseeded
- 4 tbsp olive oil
- 1 medium onion, finely chopped
- 2 cloves garlic, crushed
- 200 gr mushrooms, sliced
- 120 gr cooked millet

- 1 tbsp pine nuts (or chopped walnuts, cashew nuts or flaked almonds)
- parsley, chopped.

Preheat the oven. Clean the courgettes. Heat the oil and gently fry the onion and garlic for 2 minutes. Add the chopped mushrooms and fry a further 5 minutes. Transfer to a large bowl and add cooked millet, nuts, parsley, salt, and pepper. Stuff the courgettes "boats". Place in a baking tray, add half a cup of water and bake for 40 minutes.

Spinach and goat-cheese "quiche"

- 5 tbsp olive oil
- 500 gr spinach, trimmed and shredded
- 1 large leek, trimmed and shredded
- 1 tsp cumin seeds, lightly crushed
- 6 large pastured eggs, beaten
- 225 gr firm goat cheese, crumbled
- Salt and pepper to taste

Preheat the oven. Grease the round pie dish. Heat the oil in a large saucepan and fry the spinach, leeks and cumin seeds. Cook, stirring occasionally, for about 5 minutes, or until the vegetables have wilted and softened. Remove with a slotted spoon, transfer to a baking dish, and set aside to cool. Beat the eggs, and carefully mix in the crumbled goat's cheese. Add to the spinach. Season to taste and mix carefully. Bake for 40 minutes and let cool slightly before slicing.

Spicy fried spinach

500 gr spinach, 5 tbsp olive oil, 2 large onions, 2 cloves garlic, 1 tsp fresh ginger, 1 tsp cumin seed, ½ tsp ground coriander, 1/s tsp turmeric, ¼ tsp chili, 1 tsp salt.

Heat the oil and fry the onion, add garlic and ginger. Add seeds, ground spices, and salt, then add the spinach. Toss in the spicy mixture, turn heat very low and cook uncovered, stirring frequently until cooked. You may have to add water to prevent spinach sticking to the pan. Serve with stir-fried and cooked millet or with bread.

Desert Ideas

Wine-stewed fresh figs

- 450 ml dry white wine
- 75 gr honey
- 50 gr caster sugar
- 1 tangerine (or small orange)
- 8 whole cloves
- 450 gr fresh figs
- 1 cinnamon stick
- Fresh mint springs or bay leaves, to decorate

Put the wine, honey, and sugar in a heavy pan and heat gently, stirring constantly, until the sugar dissolves. Stud the tangerine with the coves and add to the syrup with the figs and cinnamon stick. Cover and simmer very gently for 5-10 minutes, or until the figs are softened. Transfer to a serving dish and allow to cool. Decorate the figs with mint sprigs or bay leaves.

Variation: Use fresh apricots or halved and stoned fresh peaches or nectarines in place of figs.

Raisin coconut balls

- 400 gr raisins
- 100 gr desiccated coconut

Put them in a blender or a meat-grinding machine. Make small balls. The balls taste best if made a few days in advance.

Raisin almond balls

- 75 gr raisins
- 50 gr almonds
- 50 gr coconut butter (or tahini or peanut butter)
- 25 gr shredded coconut
- Grated lemon zest (optional)

Chop the raisins in the food processor or blender to be a medium fine mixture and transfer to a bowl. Add the nuts to the food processor or blender and chop finely. Mix the nuts and raisins. Stir in the melted coconut butter (or tahini) and mix well.

Form the mixture into small balls. Roll the balls into coconut until coated.

Sesame balls

- 1 cup sesame seeds
- 1/2 cup flax seed
- 1/2 cup hazelnuts
- 2 tbsp honey
- 6-8 soft dates
- 1 tbsp coconut oil
- 1 tsp cinnamon

Grind sesame, linseed, and hazelnuts to a fine powder. Add the honey, dates, coconut oil, cinnamon and put through a food processor or a blender (alternatively, chop dates finely and knead the whole thing with your hands). Add a pinch of freshly ground nutmeg. If the mixture is too hard, you can add a little bit of water. Make small balls and serve them on dried apple slices.

<u>Variation</u>: You can use tahini, instead of coconut oil. It will have the taste of halva.

Moroccan almond biscuit fruit cups

Almond biscuits

- 1 ½ cup blanched almonds, ground
- 1 tsp baking powder
- pinch of salt
- 3 tbsp coconut butter
- 3 tbsp coconut cream

Almond filling

- 6 tbsp ground toasted almonds
- 4 tbsp caster sugar
- 1 tsp ground cinnamon

Fruit topping and glaze

- 1 mango
- 50 gr blueberries
- 50 gr red currants
- 1 tbsp lemon juice
- 1 tbsp Kirsch
- 2 tbsp caster sugar

First, make the biscuits. Preheat the oven. Line the baking dish with parchment paper. In a medium bowl combine almond flour, baking powder, and salt. Add coconut butter and press it into the flour to make it crumbly. Make a space in the middle of that mixture and crack in an egg and add the cream. With a fork, lightly mix the egg and cream together, incorporating the rest of the dough. Mix until you've formed a soft dough. Using your hands, divide dough into four pieces and roll into a ball. The dough will be soft and a bit sticky. Place dough balls onto parchment lined baking tray. DO NOT flatten dough. Bake for 20 minutes or until lightly golden. Let cool, then crumble each biscuit into a dessert dish (a glass, a cup, or a small bowl).

Prepare the almond filling by combining toasted almonds, caster sugar, and cinnamon.

To make the glazed fruits, peel the mango over a bowl, to catch the juices and cut carefully into slices with a sharp knife. To make the glaze, combine the mango juice with lemon juice, Kirsch and caster sugar in a small saucepan. Over a gentle heat, stirring constantly, cook until the sugar dissolves.

To assemble the tarts: Crumble each biscuit into a dessert dish (e.g. a glass, or a small bowl). Pour over the almond filling. Add the fruits. Spoon over a little of the fruit glaze. It tastes best if you let it stand for a couple of hours at room temperature before serving.

Pour over almond filling. Top with the fruit. Glaze.

One Last Thing!

You can help me and help others benefit from a healthy diet by leaving a review on Amazon and sharing your thoughts on this book. You have no idea how much this would help!

I also want to give you a one-in-two-hundred chance to win **a $200.00 Amazon Gift card** as a thank-you for reading this book. All I ask is that you give me some feedback, so I can improve it :)

Your opinion is super valuable to me.

It will only take a minute of your time to let me know what you like and what you didn't like about this book. The hardest part is deciding how to spend the two hundred dollars!

Just follow this link.

http://booksfor.review/ppdiet